Table of Contents

0: FRONT MATTER

Acknowledgements

I wish to extend my heartfelt thanks to all the people who have helped me in writing this book.

First to those health and nutrition experts who have inspired and educated me including:
- Clyde Wilson Ph.D., author of "What When and Water"[1]
- Stephen Phinney Ph.D. and Jeff Volek Ph.D., authors of "The Art and Science of Low Carb Performance[2]"
- Joseph Mercola D.O., author of "Fat for Fuel[3]"
- Ben Greenfield, author of "Beyond Training[4]"
- Jason Fung M.D., author of "The Obesity Code[5]"
- Mark Sisson, author of "The Primal Blueprint[6]"
- Chris Kresser M.S., L.Ac, author of "Unconventional Medicine[7]"
- Dave Asprey, author of "The Bulletproof Diet[8]"
- Eric Westman M.D. and Jimmy Moore, authors of "Keto Clarity[9]"
- Jacob Wilson M.D. and Ryan Lowery Ph.D., authors of "The Ketogenic Bible[10]"

Second to those who helped me improve this book through their thoughtful comments and corrections including:
- Abigail Romanach
- Brianna Pickering PT, DPT
- Cynthia Truelove Ph.D.

And finally, to my wife Jess who supported and tolerated my rigorous self-experimentation, walked 707 miles on the

Appalachian trail with me, tried all my recipes and never failed to give me her honest opinion of them.

About the Author

Bryan Ausinheiler is a physical therapist, personal trainer, nutritionist and author with a private telehealth practice. He is passionate about helping people improve their health and takes a science-based approach to nutrition, training and rehabilitation. His skills in searching and evaluating the research literature combined with his personal dedication to meticulous self-experimentation allow him to provide a unique perspective. He has been publishing reviews of scientific articles since 2011, first at the UCSF Synapse, and later, on his website (www.posturemovementpain.com).

About this Book

The concepts and recipes in this book will allow you to:

1. Double your body's peak fat burning rate so you can go farther, faster while getting leaner[11].
2. Cut the weight of the food in your backpack by half without cutting calories.

Your ability to burn fat will improve because of the unique metabolic changes caused by a diet high in fat, moderate in protein and very low in carbohydrates. Such a diet is called ketogenic, because it results in the conversion of fats to a form usable by the brain called ketones[10].

The ketogenic diet is not new. Ketogenic foods such as pemmican have long been used by American Indians for long distance travel. Stephen Phinney, and Jeff Volek began studying the effects of the ketogenic diet in on endurance performance in the 1980s. More recently it has begun gaining popularity in steady-state ultra-endurance events such as Ironman Triathlon and Ultra-running thanks to the work of renowned exercise physiologist Tim Noakes and its use by high profile individuals such as Ben Greenfield[4,12,13]. Many excellent ketogenic recipe books already exist, but their ingredients or techniques are unsuitable for backpacking. You are reading the first book to adapt the ketogenic diet to the specific constraints of backpacking.

The first section of this book describes the physiology of how the ketogenic diet works. When you understand the underlying mechanisms of human nutrition related to fat metabolism, especially the role of insulin, you can see how other diets that appear radically different from the ketogenic diet such as a the slow-carb diet, accomplish similar goals in different ways. This understanding will allow you to weigh the pros and cons of various dietary approaches and choose the most appropriate approach for your situation.

The second section of this book covers the details of implementing the ketogenic diet. Understanding these principles will allow you to make healthy food choices and avoid some common pitfalls.

The third section of this book covers the logistics of ketogenic backpacking.
Whether you are embarking on a 3,000 mile thru hike or just a weekend backpacking trip, this book contains everything you need to prepare and pack delicious fat-burning ketogenic meals.

The fourth section of this book contains two of my personal stories of ketogenic backpacking: 1) a 707 mile section of the Appalachian trail with my family, and 2) a two day speed-packing trip covering 51 miles and 16,913ft of elevation in the Presidential Range of the White Mountains of New Hampshire. These are true stories with meticulously collected data showing how the ketogenic diet has worked for me on the trail. I hope you find these stories both instructive and inspiring.

The fifth section of this book contains over 50 trail-tested ketogenic recipes ranging from easy meals found in resupply towns, to complex molecular gastronomy creations. Whether you are a stove-less ultra-light packer or a backcountry gourmet, the variety of flavor and texture of the recipes in this book will ensure you never get bored. You will find these recipes both delicious and easy to prepare on the trail. Even the most complex recipes in this book require nothing more than hot water and a spoon. Recipes are conveniently organized by their general flavor profile and preparation needs such as heating or a kitchen.

Each recipe includes:
1) Detailed instructions
2) Precise ingredient amounts and descriptions
3) Nutrition facts including: calories, carbohydrates, fats, proteins and Wilder ratio
4) Weight in kcal/oz
5) Cost in $/1,000 kcal
6) Estimated difficulty of preparation
7) Equipment needs
8) Recommended variations
9) Where to get hard-to-find ingredients
10) Tips for success in preparing and packing

The final section of this book contains an appendix of tables comparing recipes in this book with popular trail foods to help you plan your menu by budget or weight.

If you are not backpacking you can still use the recipes in this book to improve fat burning, endurance performance and fat loss. In fact, you may find that the convenient recipes in this book are perfectly suited to a life of frequent travel or time pressure.

Your nutritional goals and how to use this book

Stop and write down the goals for your meal plan on the trail. Now sort these goals by importance. You might have written down things like "not being hungry," "enjoying my meals," "keep from losing muscle", "feeling energetic," "optimizing my performance," "keeping my pack weight light," or "losing body fat." Keep these goals in mind as you read this book as they will influence how you use the information herein. Below are three archetypes of people I met along the Appalachian Trail and how they might use this book.

Patty Extra-Pack

Patty (trail name Extra-Pack) embarked on a flip-flop thru hike of the Appalachian Trail shortly after retiring. She had looked forward to shedding the stress of work as well as some of the extra 40+ pounds of body fat she had packed on little by little over the years. But after six weeks on the trail she was covering only 8 miles a day and was exhausted and hungry despite snacking constantly and taking breaks throughout the day. She had just weighed herself in town and was discouraged to find she had not lost any weight. It seemed like all the hiking she was doing was just increasing her appetite without burning the fat stores she had hoped to lose. Her body fat was like extra food in her pack that she couldn't eat. She was frustrated and demoralized.

Patty's inability to burn her body's fat stores was likely the result of a physiologic condition known as insulin resistance caused by years of stress, poor sleep, inactivity, a diet high in simple carbohydrates and fructose and being overweight[14]. This condition affected 57% of Americans without diabetes and 80% of those with diabetes in 2002 and its prevalence is rising[15]. When Patty consumed simple carbohydrates and her blood sugar began to rise as a result, her pancreas secreted insulin to signal the cells to take up the sugar. But her cells were insensitive to this insulin and the pancreas had to secrete a very large amount of insulin to lower her blood sugar to safe levels. Insulin reduces fat burning and this high amount of circulating insulin meant Patty could not burn her fat stores effectively [16,17].

Patty decided to do the full ketogenic diet, following the recipes in this book. Such a low carbohydrate diet has been proven to cause double the fat loss of a low-fat diet in people with insulin resistance[18]. She planned a menu from the recipes in this book incorporating sweet recipes sparingly to reduce appetite stimulation. After a tough first week of feeling lethargic, she began to feel more energetic and found she wasn't as hungry and didn't feel the urge to snack anymore. Three weeks later she was covering 14 miles a day and had lost five pounds. She went on to successfully complete her hike and lose over 30 pounds.

Insatiable Candy Andy

Andy (trail name Candy Andy), had just entered the White Mountains of New Hampshire on a northbound attempt on the Appalachian Trail and was pushing for 25+ miles a day to finish during his summer break from college. He was famous for consuming a steady supply of candy throughout the day and was hungry and getting hungrier. Every time he opened his food bag it took all his willpower to stop himself from eating its entire contents. If he loaded up his pack with food his shin splits immediately let him know about it, but if he went light on food he felt famished and slow after one day back on the trail in a way that gorging in town never seemed to make up for.

Although Andy eats large amounts of refined carbohydrates, he is highly active and young, and his dietary choices have yet to catch up with him. He secretes less insulin when eating carbohydrates than Patty because his muscle takes up some of the blood sugar and he is much more insulin sensitive. As a result, he can eat simple carbohydrates, even sugar, with a less profound reduction in his ability to burn fat than Patty. But his current diet of jelly beans, snickers, energy bars, peanut butter wraps and ramen noodles both prevents him from achieving his maximal fat burning capacity and would be too heavy to carry if he brought as many calories as he was burning. With his current menu, 5,000kcal/day would weigh 4lbs.

Andy had to make a choice to go for the full ketogenic diet with severe carbohydrate restriction and moderate protein to ensure a full metabolic shift to fat burning, or to simply add more fat on top of his current menu to get more calories with the least possible additional weight.

He chose the second option, and added butter to his peanut butter wraps, and coconut oil to his oatmeal and ramen. This "add more fat to your carbs" strategy would have been disastrous for Patty as the high carb intake plus her insulin resistance would shunt these extra fats to storage and then prevent them from being released, but for young Andy who was insulin sensitive and running a severe caloric deficit, this strategy knocked out his hiker hunger almost overnight.

Initially he was concerned that the expense of coconut oil would put him over budget, but he found that per calorie many fats and oils were more affordable than he expected

14

albeit not as cheap as honey buns (see appendix). In the end, he more than recouped his investment in healthy oils by spending less at restaurants in town.

After some initial trouble digesting the extra coconut oil (nothing as bad as some of his post town day binges) he found himself markedly less hungry with the addition of only 1/2lb of fat to his daily food bag.

Muscle Matt

Matt was 33 years old, an avid cross-fitter and strict follower of the Mark Sisson's Primal Blueprint diet[6]. When several of his old friends from college started trying to convince him to join them for a thru hike of the Pacific Crest Trail (PCT) he was concerned that the combination of chronic cardio, no weight-lifting and caloric restriction would result in him losing muscle and high intensity performance. He wasn't sure what exactly he would eat and recognized how ironically challenging it is to eat paleo while backpacking. In theory, living outdoors would naturally fit with the paleo diet but if you spend all day hiking instead of hunting, fishing and foraging you are left trying to survive on jerky or eating processed long shelf-life foods that are rarely paleo friendly.

When Matt discovered ketogenic backpacking, he was particularly interested in the lean-mass sparing effects of low-carbohydrate calorie-sufficient diets[11,19,20]. When ketones are present in the bloodstream, they are used for fuel instead of branched chain amino acids thus sparing muscle breakdown that would otherwise occur to provide these amino acids[21,22]. Dirk did weekly body weight strength workouts consisting of pullups, handstand pushups and single leg squats during rest days off the trail. He also supplemented with branched chain amino acids on the trail as extra insurance after he heard about a study that found they helped preserve lean mass during caloric restriction[23,24]tevia. He started the ketogenic diet eight weeks before the hike and had little trouble adapting and finding which meals he liked the best. In the first few weeks on the ketogenic diet he noticed a dip in his performance on many of the shorter Crossfit benchmark workouts such as Amanda and Grace but improved his time in the longer slogs like Murph, but by the end of eight weeks he had improved all of his benchmark workouts[125]. He ended up hiking the entire PCT with his friends and when he returned to the gym five and a half months later he was a few pounds lighter and noticeably weaker in the heavy lifts but could do more pullups than ever before. But after a few months in the gym he was back to his prior level of fitness and felt the ketogenic backpacking food played a crucial role in reducing muscle loss on the trail.

---

[1] Rachel Gregory of James Madison University investigated the effects of a ketogenic diet on performance in 27 non-elite cross fit athletes and found similar improvements in performance as the control group.

KETOGENIC BACKPACKING

Pack Lighter and Go Farther by Fueling with Fat
by Bryan Ausinheiler PT,DPT,CSCS,OCS,FNS

I: UNDERSTANDING THE KETOGENIC DIET

1. What is a ketogenic diet and why is it ideal for backpacking?

A diet that is extremely low in carbohydrates, adequate but moderate in protein and high in fat is called a ketogenic diet because on this diet the liver converts fat into ketones to fuel the brain and body[2,10].

A ketogenic diet has several advantages for backpacking:

1. **Eating a ketogenic diet improves your ability to burn fat.** If you do not effectively burn fat on a diet containing carbohydrates, the ability to burn fat can be twice as high on a ketogenic diet[11]. This means an efficient use of both body fat and ingested fat for a constant energy supply during long, moderate to low intensity endurance activity such as hiking. Even if you are lean you are likely to have 10lbs of non-essential fat containing 30,000kcal, which is enough to fuel a 155lb (70kg) person for 55 hours of backpacking with a light pack covering 109 miles at 2mph[26]. In comparison, the maximum carbohydrate stores of even the most elite athletes is 2,000kcal which would be depleted after only 3.7 hours of backpacking covering only 7.3 miles at 2mph[2,26].

2. **Ketogenic meals can be half the weight of conventional backpacking meals.** This is in addition to lightening your body weight by burning fat stored on your body.

3. **In theory, a ketogenic diet would allow for a more rapid recovery from prolonged exercise** because it has been shown to have lower systemic inflammation levels than a high carbohydrate diet[27]. In addition to causing inflammation, exercise causes damage to cell membranes through the formation of free radicals known as reactive

oxygen species. The ketogenic diet may be protective against this stress as ketone infusions have been shown to protect against oxidative stress in rat brains and ketogenic diets in humans have found either favorable changes or no change on reactive oxygen species and antioxidant levels[28-31]. However, there are many variables that effect the production and neutralization of reactive oxygen species and the net effect of the ketogenic diet is still unclear[32].

4. The ketogenic diet is your ultimate weapon against "hiker hunger" caused by inadequate caloric intake for several reasons: 1) Ketogenic meals are so much lighter per calorie than other backpacking foods that you can carry and eat almost twice as many calories for the same pack weight. 2) The high energy density of fats allows you to eat a lot of calories in a short period of time with little chewing. This fact that can lead to overeating and weight gain in the sedentary individual but can help a 10-hour-per-day speed-packer get the extra 5,460kcal they need to maintain their body weight that they would be otherwise too tired to chew. Studies consistently show adding more fat to high carbohydrate foods (yogurt and muffins) results in people eating more calories at that meal without reducing their intake at the following meal[33,34]. The effects on satiation and satiety of ketogenic foods with sweetened with non-caloric sweeteners such as those in this has not been investigated but I suspect it to be similar. 3) Burning fat reduces hunger between meals (increased satiety) through a variety of mechanisms including inhibiting the hormone ghrelin[34]. This is especially true of medium chain triglycerides which have been shown to reduce appetite[34]. Despite the fact that meals that result in greater insulin secretion (carbohydrates and protein) result in a greater feeling of fullness, as a whole, ketogenic diets have been shown to result in lower hunger levels[35,36]. If your hunger is not the result of inadequate caloric intake, increasing your intake of fiber is the smartest way to impact satiation and satiety[37].

2. The Basis Mechanics of Metabolism and Ketosis

Your body can extract energy from the chemical bonds found in fat, carbohydrates, protein and alcohol. The first three of these are known as "macronutrients" because they are consumed in large quantities compared to micronutrients like vitamins and minerals. Each macronutrient follows a maze of different metabolic pathways that vary according to the ratio of macronutrients consumed, the intensity of physical activity and hormonal factors influenced by age, gender, stress and genetic variation[38].

The human metabolism system is very complex but there are several key facts you should know when embarking on a ketogenic diet.

1) The highest priority of your metabolic system is to fuel your brain.
2) Your brain can only burn two types of fuel: glucose and ketones.
3) Your brain has no substantial store of these energy sources and relies on a constant supply of them in the blood stream.
4) Blood glucose can be supplied by the carbohydrates you ate in the last few hours, your body's carbohydrate stores (glycogen) and/or made from the glycerol component of far or from dietary protein or protein scavenged from the body's tissues.
5) Blood ketones are supplied from recently eaten fats or your body's fat stores but are only produced by

the liver when its own carbohydrate (glycogen) stores are depleted.

6) Eating carbohydrates and protein stimulate the secretion of the hormone insulin which reduces your ability to release stored fat to be burned for 36 hours.

7) If enough carbohydrates are consumed to prevent the production of ketones (usually >50g/day) but not enough to fuel your brain and muscle (usually <150g/day), blood glucose supply can be compromised especially during intense activity and mental and physical performance will suffer.

8) **For this reason, I strongly recommend either committing fully to the ketogenic to ensure the production of ketones or eating adequate carbohydrates to maintain stable blood glucose**

Why Ketones Matter

Ketones matter because they fuel your brain when carbohydrates are scarce, and a well fueled brain is a happy, well-functioning brain. A ketogenic diet is a diet that shifts your body towards using fat for fuel in the form of ketones. This diet consists of carbohydrate restriction and moderate protein intake according to the level your body needs to produce ketones. A ketogenic diet may also include highly ketogenic foods such as medium chain triglycerides and exogenous ketones.

On the other hand, a low carbohydrate diet simply describes a diet arbitrarily low in carbohydrate which is often high in protein and may or may not result in nutritional ketosis. If you can lose weight and/or feel energetic on a low carb diet without producing ketones, then don't worry about the ketones. You are either burning fat efficiently, readily synthesize sufficient glucose from lactate, glycerol and protein, and/or your exercise intensity is very low. However, a risk of a low carb but non-ketogenic diet is that you will feel periodically weak and/or cognitively impaired due to low blood glucose and glycogen stores without ketones present as an alternative fuel for the brain, muscles and organs. These side effects are especially likely in the context of prolonged exertion such as backpacking. It is for this reason that I focus on ketone production as opposed to carbohydrate restriction per se.

Measurable blood ketone levels are a reliable sign that your brain and body are being fueled by fat. In studies on rodents, when blood ketone (beta-hydroxybutyrate) levels are 1mmol/dl, 50% of the brain's energy is supplied by ketones[39]. The brain peaks at 75% ketone use as the remaining neurons are only able to metabolize glucose[40,41]. On a ketogenic diet this remaining glucose is supplied by a combination of dietary carbohydrates and glucose manufactured in the liver from byproducts such as lactate and pyruvate as well as protein and fat (specifically the glycerol backbone of triglycerides)[42]. During a prolonged fast, 67% of the brain's energy comes from ketones, 17% from glucose made from lactate and pyruvate, 8% from glucose made from fat (the glycerol backbone of triglycerides) and 8% from glucose made from protein.

The ability to produce ketones is a critical survival skill that allows us humans to go long periods without eating by converting stored body fat into energy useable the brain. When compared to other animals, we are both uniquely good at getting fat and at producing ketones. These abilities probably have something to do with the primary importance of fueling our large energy-hungry brains. Our babies are standouts in this regard. They are born incredibly fat at 15% body fat, compared to other primates that are born at <4% fat. A human newborn spends 75% of their energy on brain growth and metabolism and produces ketones from birth. These ketone bodies provide 25% of calories in the first few days of life[43].

When does your liver make ketones?

On a mixed diet, the liver burns fat via a process called the citric acid cycle. Oxaloacetate is primarily derived from carbohydrates and is a key step in the citric acid cycle. When the amount of fat being delivered to the liver to be burned is greater than the amount of oxaloacetate available to run the citric acid cycle, the remaining fat is converted into ketones[44].

Thus, one way to stimulate ketone production is to let your liver run out of its carbohydrate stores (glycogen). Oxaloacetate is then used to create blood sugar through gluconeogenesis and is quickly depleted[45]. This can occur in as little as a day of fasting or two days on a ketogenic diet[41,46].

There are many other mechanisms that regulate your ketone production but a major one is the storage signaling hormone insulin. A spike in insulin caused by rapidly digested carbohydrates or animal protein stops the release of fat from fat cells and thus less fat is delivered to the liver for metabolism and ketone production is reduced[47,48].

How Fat Intake Effects Ketosis

Technically, you don't need to eat fat to make ketones, you only need to avoid carbohydrates and protein. In fact, blood ketone levels of 5mmol/L are consistently found during 3-5 weeks of eating nothing at all[49,50]. This is because the hormone glucagon is signaling the body's fat stores to be released and sent to the liver which has depleted its carbohydrates stores[41].

Prolonged fasting is a reliable way to burn body fat and produce ketones but unsurprisingly it impairs endurance performance[51]. Fasting every other day results in less of a drop in basal metabolic rate and lean mass than daily caloric restriction and thus may be an effective way to reduce body fat and maintain that lower weight in the long term[52,53]. Periodic fasting for weight loss is increasingly advocated by health professionals among the most prominent of which is Dr Jason Fung, author of "The Obesity Code"[5]. However, fasting may be better suited to lose weight before starting a long-distance hike as the combination of hiking and fasting greatly increases the risk of impaired performance.

Eating fat supplies immediate energy for the body and brain and elevates ketone levels faster than fasting. Eating a lot of fat at once with very little carbohydrate and moderate protein is especially effective at producing ketones because this large amount of fat easily overwhelms the scanty amount of oxaloacetate present in the liver and little insulin is secreted to signal the fat to be stored.

How Protein Intake Effects Ketosis

High protein foods such as meat, fish and eggs stimulate the secretion of insulin directly and insulin inhibits ketone production[47]. When carbohydrates are absent and dietary protein intake is >30% of calories, protein can be converted to blood glucose at a rate sufficient to refill the liver's glycogen stores[54]. Full liver glycogen stores will prevent ketone production[2,44]. Without ketone production the brain will be entirely dependent on blood sugar for fuel and thus at risk of energy shortages during intense exercise. Furthermore, when protein intake exceeds the amount needed for bodily repair and blood glucose levels are normal, the remainder is stored as fat.

Excessive protein intake will stall ketone production by being used as a substrate to make oxaloacetate and by stimulating insulin secretion, but a moderate protein intake is necessary on a ketogenic diet for several reasons[2].

First, some proteins contain branched chain amino acids which can be metabolized by the muscle directly as a supplemental fuel during prolonged and intense endurance activity[55]. This reliance on protein as fuel has been shown to increase with the depletion of glycogen stores, and when you are eating a ketogenic diet you are constantly in a glycogen depleted state[56]. The branched chain amino acids are leucine, isoleucine and valine and are found in all complete protein sources[44].

Second, adequate protein intake is necessary to maintain muscle mass[57]. Although the presence of ketones in the blood stream will reduce the breakdown of muscle for fuel, protein intake is still required as muscle and other lean mass is constantly recycled and replaced[57].

The ketogenic diet and muscle mass

Will you lose or gain muscle on a ketogenic diet? The answer is not that much different than it would be on any diet, if you do resistance training and eat adequate protein you will gain muscle, if you stop resistance training or don't eat sufficient protein or calories you will lose muscle.

Your risk of losing muscle mass is highest if you are severely cutting calories without adequate protein.

In theory a reduced calorie ketogenic diet would put you at a high risk of losing muscle mass because it results in low insulin levels. Insulin plays an important role in both fat storage and muscle building and insulin has a protective effect on body muscle. When insulin levels are low due to carbohydrate restriction, cortisol is released which increases muscle and fat break down, but ketones are produced which reduce muscle breakdown.

Although low insulin should make it hard to gain muscle on a ketogenic diet several studies have shown similar gains in muscle mass on ketogenic (<50g of carbohydrates per day) and low fat (<25% of calories as fat) diets with greater loss of body fat in the low carbohydrate group[19,57]. When eating sufficient calories and a moderate protein intake, the ketogenic diet does not result in a loss of lean body mass.

If you are severely restricting your caloric intake on the ketogenic diet while thru-hiking in an attempt to lose a large amount of body fat, you are at risk of losing lean mass as well. With a few exceptions, most studies on the use of the ketogenic diet for weight loss shows that very low carbohydrate and moderate protein diets preserves lean body mass just as well if not better than a low-fat diet with the same caloric debt[58-63]. Even severe caloric restriction (~800kcal/day) and very mild ketosis has been shown to result in fat loss with minimal loss of muscle when protein intake was 0.8-1.2g/kg of ideal (not actual) body weigh[59]. Keep in mind that none of these studies were conducted on people hiking 8 hours a day, an activity that is likely to result in more muscle loss due to the high energy demand.

If you are concerned about losing muscle on a thru hike, I recommend one day of strength training per week and a protein intake at or above 0.8g/kg of body weight if you are eating sufficient calories, and higher if you are in a caloric deficit.

Although strength and muscle mass are related, they are not the same thing. Strength is a product of both muscle mass and the ability to use it and the nervous system plays an equal if not greater role in strength than does muscle size. A seminal eastern-bloc study on detraining demonstrated maintenance of strength for up to 30 days without training in individuals with a long history of strength training[64]. On a thru-hike supplemented with strength training it is possible to lose some muscle mass while maintaining strength and this is ideal for sports in which strength to weight ratio is paramount.

3. Other Options: Maximizing Fat Metabolism Without Going Ketogenic.

The ketogenic diet isn't for everyone but fortunately it isn't the only way to maximize your body's ability to burn fat. If you would like to increase fat burning and feel energetic without the careful carbohydrate and protein monitoring needed to achieve ketosis there are still a few things you can do and they all revolve around keeping insulin levels low and improving insulin sensitivity.

1) **Eat slow carbs and avoid fast carbs.** Avoid quick-digesting carbohydrates including sugar, pastries, bread, rice, pasta, starchy tubers and non-fibrous fruits as these impair fat burning[65,66]. Instead consume slow-digesting minimally processed, non-starchy whole plants to keep your body's glycogen stores full (at least 370g/day for small athletes and 500g/day for large athletes in training[44]).

2) **Eat good fats.** Consume sufficient fat to supply remaining energy needs from sources that reduce inflammation and increase fat burning including omega-3 rich fish oil, olive, avocado and coconut oil, grass fed butter and medium chain triglycerides[67,68].

3) **Feed your gut microbes** with generous amounts of fiber and resistant starch[69].

To eat a slow-carb diet while backpacking, take the recipes in this book as a starting point and increase or add generous amounts of freeze dried or dehydrated vegetables.

Why Speed of Carbohydrate Digestion Matters

All carbohydrates, from broccoli to skittles are eventually broken down in the intestines into the building blocks of sugar called monosaccharides. There are three monosaccharides: glucose, fructose and galactose. All carbohydrates become monosaccharides, but the speed in which this happens varies greatly between foods and has a major impact on how your body stores and uses energy.

"Fast carbs" include the monosaccharides themselves (glucose, fructose and galactose) as well as simple combinations of these including table sugar: sucrose (glucose plus fructose), and milk sugar: lactose (glucose plus galactose).

Besides sugar, other quick digesting carbohydrates include any carbohydrates that are not bound to fiber or have been highly processed. This includes all cooked modern agricultural grains and tubers as they have been selectively bred for millennia to have as much sugar and as little fiber as possible. Processes such as milling and grinding further separates the starch from the fiber and break plants down into very small pieces that are easily digested.

"Fast Carbs" includes sugar, candies, pastries, bread, rice, pasta, oatmeal, cream of wheat, grits, cooked root vegetables such as potatoes, yams, yucca, beets and carrots and low-fiber or dried fruits such as dates and raisins.

The effect of food processing on weight gain has been demonstrated with a clever by Desmarchelier et al. who fed identical standard chow to two groups of mice but to one group it was given in the form of hard pellets and in the other it was given in the form of soft flour. The mice fed the flour form became obese while the others did not[70]. The health of a food is not intrinsic to an ingredient but is largely influenced by the amount of processing and refinement it undergoes.

"Slow carbs" are broken down into monosaccharides slowly because it takes your digestive system a long time to disassemble the long carbohydrate chains and disentangle them from the fiber and parts of the plant that you ate[71].

Once carbohydrates are broken down into monosaccharides, they enter the blood stream. When you measure your blood sugar with a finger prick test you are monitoring the monsaccharide glucose. Fasting blood glucose levels over 100mg/dL are dangerous as the sugar literally causes damage to your blood vessels through physical shear and damage to the kidneys, eyes and other areas through glycosylation with damaging increasing as blood sugar levels rise further[72,73]. Elevated blood glucose damage causes inflammation and increases your risk of a host of diseases from diabetes to heart disease and even cancer[73-75].

To prevent blood sugar from rising too high after a meal, your pancreas secretes a hormone called insulin which signals cells throughout the body, including fat cells, to take sugar out of the blood and store it as fat. Insulin also stops your fat cells from releasing their fat stores by binding and inactivating hormone-sensitive lipase[2].

The faster glucose enters your bloodstream from your digestive tract, the more insulin your pancreas must secrete to get it under control. High levels of insulin inhibit fat burning and increase the risk of becoming insulin resistant resulting in ever higher levels of insulin and greater difficulty burning fat[76].

Thus, to maximize fat burning insulin levels must be low most of the time. At the time of this writing, technology does not exist for continuous personal insulin monitoring so there is no objective way for you to precisely calibrate your meals to control your insulin response. There is large variation between people in the amount of insulin secreted following any given meal[77]. Without knowing your individual response, it is best to be safe and avoid sugar and other quick-digesting carbohydrates.

Good Fats Burn Fat

If you eat a food high in both quick digesting carbohydrates and fat (i.e. a donut), the carbs are burned while the fat is stored directly, and fat burning is reduced. Research studies demonstrating the fattening effects of a "high fat diet" invariable use a diet higher in quick digesting carbs (~50%) than fat (~40%). Fat has been blamed for the fattening effect because it is what get stored, even though it's the carbs that make it so hard to burn off the stored fat.

There are two types of fat that promote fat burning directly, namely omega-3 fatty acids and medium chain triglycerides.

The list of health benefits of omega-3 fatty acids is wide reaching. There are mechanisms by which omega-3 fatty acids stimulate fat burning by: stimulating leptin secretion, improve insulin sensitivity, improving glycogen storage, reducing fat storage, facilitating transport of fatty acids into the cell for metabolism and reducing fat cell inflammation[78,79]. Test your blood levels of omega-3 with the Holman Blood test then increase your intake of cold water fatty fish such as sardines and salmon or consume a fresh, high quality fish oil supplement and test again to ensure adequate levels and an equal omega-3/omega-6 ratio. The amount of omega-3 you need to eat will be unique to you as each person metabolizes omega-3s at different rates.

Medium chain triglycerides (MCTs) are more easily burned for immediate energy than other fats because they do not require carnitine to enter your cells and they depend to a lesser extent on fatty acid binding proteins[80]. MCTs can be turned into ketone bodies even when carbohydrates are not severely restricted[81]. MCTs are found in coconut oil and to a lesser extent butter and can also be extracted and consumed directly. See more on MCTs in the "gut health" chapter of this book as overconsumption can lead to severe gastrointestinal discomfort.

Feed Your Microbiome

The health benefits of dietary fiber are wide reaching and well documented from decreased risk of cardiovascular disease, obesity and cancer[82-84]. Fiber comes in many forms including arabinoxylan, inulin, pectin, bran, cellulose, β-glucan and resistant starch. Some fiber passes through your intestines without being digested by your or your gut microbes but nonetheless slows your absorption of carbohydrates and thus reduces your insulin spike even when added as a supplement to a meal[82]. Other fibers feed your gut microbes and are called fermentable fibers. These include prebiotics and resistant starch.

Resistant starch is starch that resists direct digestion but is subsequently digested by the bacteria in your large intestine. Your bacteria then convert some of the starch to free fatty acids that are the preferred fuel of your intestinal cells and provide you with energy several hours after the meal. This round-about way of eating has been found to have a host of health benefits[85-87]. Replacing 5% of the carbohydrates in a meal with resistant starch was found to increase fat metabolism by 23%[88]. Consuming 30 grams of resistant starch per day improved insulin sensitivity by 33% in healthy individuals and 40 grams a day improved insulin sensitivity by 16% in people with insulin resistance[89,90]. Resistant starch is most plentiful in raw potatoes and green bananas. Raw potato starch and green banana flour can be easily brought on the trail and mixed into meals. Note that resistant starch is only resistant to digestion when raw, once cooked it is digested as quickly as any dense carbohydrate.

4. Is the ketogenic diet right for you?

If your goal is weight loss, both a low carb and a slow-carb diet have been shown equally effective, and both are significantly more effective than a low-fat diet[18,91]. If your goal is enjoyment, this will vary by your preferences. Do you love or loath the idea of putting lard on salami? If your goal is reducing pack weight and food prep time, the ketogenic diet is a clear winner.

While the ketogenic diet can be frustratingly difficult to implement while traveling and eating out, it is quite easy to do on a long-distance backpacking trip if you packed all your meals in advance. In fact, the ketogenic diet can be easy and simple for someone who can tolerate low variety. Conversely, a slow-carb diet consisting of minimally processed plants and wild animals is extremely healthy and not terribly hard to do when refrigeration is available but is difficult if not impossible to do while backpacking. Hiking all day doesn't leave time for hunting and gathering, and fresh produce and meats are heavy to carry and don't keep well on the trail. Fiber contains practically no calories at all, and dehydrated or freeze dried fibrous vegetables are proportionally heavy, bulky and expensive for the small number of calories they provide, not to mention time consuming to cook. You may find a slow-carb approach quite manageable if you don't need to eat a lot because you are averaging 8 miles per day and have extra body fat to burn. But if you have a high metabolism, little stored body fat and are doing big miles, a slow carb diet will be nearly impossible on the trail.

Remember, if you choose to eat carbs, eat them regularly. Very few people have the metabolic flexibility to cycle in and out of ketosis without experiencing detrimental effects on their mental or physical performance.

II. EATING THE KETOGENIC DIET

5. How to Get into Ketosis

Getting into ketosis is simple, just eat all your meals from this book and I guarantee you will be in ketosis within six weeks as measured by blood beta-hydroxybutyrate levels >1mmol/L one hour after a meal.

There are several different strategies to enter nutritional ketosis without fasting 1) The Wilder Ratio, 2) Carbohydrate and Protein Limits, and 3) Medium Chain Triglycerides Supplementation.

The macro nutrient requirement to enter ketosis is simple:

> Eat >3 grams of fat for every 1 gram of combined carbohydrates and protein at every meal.

This ratio of grams of fat divided by combined grams of protein carbohydrates is called the Wilder ratio. All the recipes in this book have a Wilder ratio of 3 or greater. To make a Wilder Ratio of 3:1, a meal with 5 grams of carbs and 10 grams of protein would need to be accompanied by

45 grams of fat. You will need to check food labels and weigh and measure all your food for several days if you are making meals outside of this cookbook. I recommend getting comfortable making several ketogenic meals that you like before embarking on the diet.

The Wilder Ratio isn't the only way to adjust macronutrients to get into ketosis. If you prefer to only track carbohydrates and protein, then eat as much fat as needed to feel full and:

1) Limit carbohydrates to <30g/day spread out throughout the day. None of which should come from simple carbohydrates (sugar, starch, bread, rice, pasta, pastries etc.). People with lower daily caloric needs may have to limit carbohydrate intake to as little as 10g/day.

2) Limit protein to 0.36-1.0g of protein per pound of body weight spread out throughout the day.

You can also produce ketones with little to no carbohydrate or protein restriction by consume large amounts of MCT oil. This will certainly produce ketones to fuel your brain and body but will do little to improve your peak fat burning rate and runs a high risk of gastrointestinal symptoms.

It is important to note that *simply adding more fat to a moderate or high carbohydrate diet will not result in ketosis because to produce ketones the liver must be depleted of stored carbohydrates (glycogen).* Liver carbohydrate depletion occurs in <48 hours on a ketogenic diet and can occur in <12 hours with a ketogenic diet is combined with intense exercise[41,46].

Eating a high protein, high fat diet is unlikely to result in ketosis because if protein intake is high, gluconeogenesis can keep liver glycogen full indefinitely.

However, if protein intake is moderate, the liver will begin to turn fat into ketones that fuel the brain, muscles and organs. A moderate protein intake ranges between a lower limit of 0.30 grams of protein per pounds of body weight (estimated to meet the needs of 50% of the population) up to 1 gram per pound of body weight recommended by ketogenic researchers Stephen Phinney and Jeff Volek[2,92]. Phinney and Volek recommend the higher protein intake for athletes to offset protein burned during prolonged and intense exercise in the form of branched chain amino acids. I personally found that a higher protein intake severely reduced ketone production and you can read more about my experience in the "Keto on The Trail" section of this book. Ketone production increased when I reduced my protein to Dr. Mercola's recommendation of 1-1.25g or protein per kilogram of lean body mass[3]. To make this calculation you will need an accurate body composition assessment such as a DEXA scan.

Summary of various protein recommendations.
- 0.30g/lb/day (0.66g/kg/day): The Estimated Average Requirement (EAR) of the Institute of Medicine of the US National Academy of Sciences[93].
- 0.36g/lb/day (0.80g/kg/day): The Recommended Dietary Allowance (RDA) of the Institute of Medicine of the US National Academy of Sciences[93].
- 1-1.25g/lb of lean mass/day (2.2-2.75g/lb of lean mass/day): Recommendation of natural health expert Dr. Joseph Mercola[3].
- 1.0g/lb/day (2.2g/kg/day): Recommended by ketogenic diet researches Stephen Phinney and Jeff Volek[2].

My advice: To optimize fat metabolism, endurance performance and reduce cancer risk: start at the lowest protein intake and gradually increase to the highest protein intake at which blood ketones are still >1mmol. To optimize building or maintaining muscle mass: increase protein intake to the highest level at which your energy levels remain constant and your pack weight not overly burdensome.

6. A Guide to Healthy Fats

You may be wondering if a diet consisting of 90% fat is healthy. The answer is yes only if the fats themselves are healthy. The low-fat diet craze that started with Senator McGovern's hearing on diet and heart disease in 1976 labeled all fats as unhealthy and the very first dietary guidelines that came out as a result recommended a reduction in all fat intake[3,94]. As a proportion of calories, America's fat intake did decrease in the following decades as people chose lower-fat options, but their total caloric intake increased so much that the absolute value of fat was still higher 2010 than 1970, particularly in vegetable oil[95]. The advice to reduce fat, replace saturated fat with vegetable oil and increase carbohydrate intake was ineffective as obesity, heart disease, diabetes and cancer continued to rise. The Women's Health Initiative Dietary Modification Trial of 48,835, the largest randomized controlled trial of its kind, failed to find weight loss or health benefits from reducing total dietary fat intake from 38% to 29% of calories[96-99]. The effects of ketogenic diets on blood lipids has been studied and a frequent finding of lowered triglycerides and elevated high density lipoprotein (HDL) and either stable or elevated low-density lipoprotein (LDL) has been found[83,100-102]. The relevance of cholesterol as a marker of cardiovascular health has been challenged, as elevated cholesterol levels seem less important than whether there is inflammation in the blood vessels that will stimulate the deposition of this cholesterol in plaque[103]. "Furthermore, ketogenic diets increase the size of LDL particles resulting in fewer of the more dangerous (atherosclerotic) small particles[104].

However, not all studies on the health effects of low carbohydrate (not necessarily ketogenic) diets have been positive, as several have found a stiffening of the blood vessel walls, increases in markers of inflammation and increase risk of all-cause mortality (although not cardiovascular disease)[100,105,106]. As these studies did not control for omega-3 and omega-6 consumption, protein intake, ketone levels or exposure to oxidized fats, it is not clear if these effects are the result of a low-carb diet rich in unhealthy fats or if these effects are inherent to low-carbohydrate diets.

Cholesterol

Cholesterol plays many important roles in the body. Hormones such as testosterone and estrogen are made of cholesterol, as is 20% of the insulin of your nerve cells (myelin). A high carbohydrate, high fructose and low cholesterol diet has been linked to the development of Alzheimer's disease[107]. Fatty animal products are rich in cholesterol and a ketogenic diet that includes them is likely to be high in cholesterol. Your body can synthesize most of the cholesterol it needs, and your blood cholesterol levels are most strongly influenced by this synthesis. Should you try to limit your intake of cholesterol rich foods? The 2015 report from the Dietary Guidelines Advisory Committee of the US Department of Public Health declared "cholesterol is not considered a nutrient of concern for overconsumption.[108]"

Saturated, Unsaturated and Trans Fat

A fatty acid consists of a long chain of carbon atoms with hydrogen atoms bound to each side. In a saturated fat, all the carbon sites are full of hydrogen atoms. In a monounsaturated fat, one of the carbon sites is missing a hydrogen atom and as a result it forms a double bond to the adjacent carbon. In a polyunsaturated fat, there are numerous locations where hydrogen atoms are missing, and double bonds of carbon are formed.

Saturated fats are more likely to be solid at room temperature and make up a large percentage of animal fats.

Except for coconut and palm oil, vegetable oils are comprised of unsaturated fat that are liquid at room temperature. In 1902 Wilhelm Normann invented the process of hydrogenation which adds hydrogen atoms to the unsaturated fats to turn them into saturated fats. When the hydrogen atoms are bound to the same side of the carbon atom they repel each other and bend the chain thus preventing the chains from packing in tightly. This same-side binding is called the called the "cis" position and is found in some natural unsaturated fats. If the hydrogen atoms are on opposite sides, in the "trans" position they balance each other and straighten the chain thus allowing the chains to pack tightly. The "trans" position is found in hydrogenated oils and thus they are called "trans fats." Hydrogenation turned vegetable oils into shortening with all the wonderful textural properties of saturated fats coveted by bakers for making flaky crusts and moist pastries at a fraction of the cost of animal fats like butter.

Unfortunately, the effects of hydrogenated trans fats on health have been disastrous. It took several decades for science to find the fly in the ointment of hydrogenated fats but the results are now conclusive. Hydrogenated "trans" fats promote inflammation and their consumption is detrimental to health and should be avoided[109,110]. As affordable and ketogenic as it might be, you won't find Crisco in any of the recipes in this book.

Trans-fat is dangerous, but what about non-hydrogenated sources of saturated fat? An enormous systematic review including 530,525 people from around the world failed to find a link between saturated fat intake and cardiovascular health, although they did find that omega-3 from fatty fish had a protective effect[111]. In addition, the Sydney Diet Heart Study randomly assigned 458 men to either a control group or an intervention group that was given unsaturated fats high in omega-6 in the form of margarine and safflower oils to replace their saturated fat intake in an attempt to improve their health[112]. The result was that after 10 years, the death rate was 18% in the group receiving the omega-6 from vegetable oils vs 12% in the control group[112].

Omega 3 and Omega 6

Among the unsaturated fatty acids, there are several which the body critically needs but cannot construct from other fatty acids and thus are considered essential fatty acids. There are two essential unsaturated fatty acids, named omega 3 and omega 6 because the missing hydrogen atom is 3 carbons and 6 carbons from the "omega" tail end of the chain respectively.

Omega 3 and Omega 6 fatty acids are critical building blocks in numerous biological functions, most notably the formation of inflammatory precursors called eicosanoids. Omega 3 fatty acids are made into eicosanoids that reduce and control inflammation while omega 6 fatty acids are made into eicosanoids that promote inflammation. Both are necessary, but the balance of Omega 3 and 6 in the diet influences the amount of each type of eicosanoid produced and tips the system either toward or away from inflammation[67,68,113].

The list of benefits from omega-3 fatty acid consumption is astounding[78,113,114]. The results are most consistently positive in studies that measure blood levels of omega-3 and omega-6 as individuals vary in absorption rates and the presence of high quantities of omega-6 in the diet can negate omega-3 supplementation.

Omega 3 fatty acids are found plentifully in fatty fish and aquatic mammals, krill oil and to a smaller extant are present in wild game and pasture fed animals, insects and eggs. In these sources, omega 3 is present in the form of DHA (docosahexaenoic acid) and EPA (eicosapentaenoic acid) which directly used to produce anti-inflammatory eicosanoids.

Omega-3 fatty acids can also be derived from breaking down alpha linoleic acid found in plant sources such as chia, flax and hemp seeds, walnuts and leafy greens. However only about 1% of ALA is converted into the omega-3 EPA and none into DHA. Conversion is particularly poor if omega-6 intake is high as ALA and omega-6 compete for the same enzymes and thus typical vegetarian sources of omega-3 are unable to balance the omega-3/omega-6 ratio[115]. Several studies have found micro-algae oil supplementation increases blood DHA and this is a promising area of research for vegetarians[115].

Rancidification and Contamination

Although a bag of olive oil will keep fresh longer on the trail than a box of pastries, it won't last forever and as it becomes rancid it will not only lose its healthy properties but will become harmful. This is a major concern on long distance through hikes when one is shipping food ahead that may sit in a warm post office for months.

Rancidification refers to the process by which fats are broken down and produce unpleasant odors or flavors. This is more than just a concern for flavor, as experimental data in animals has shown rancid oils show up in the bloodstream and cause inflammation. Data in humans has correlated the consumption of rancid oils with inflammatory diseases and blood vessel damage (atherosclerosis)[116].

These effects have been found in diets consisting of only moderate fat intake, and for someone eating a ketogenic diet consisting of 90% fat, fat rancidification should be a major concern.

Fat can become rancid from any combination of contact with the following[117]:
  1. Oxygen (oxidative rancidity)
  2. Water (hydrolytic rancidity)
  3. Microbes (microbial rancidity).

Heat increase the rate of rancidification by all three mechanisms and light speeds up the rate of oxidative rancidification.

Initially, the flavor and odor changes of rancidification are subtle, and the first step of oxidative rancidification, called "activation" often goes without notice. Even as rancidification progresses, many people will not be able to detect the changes, as rancidity initially decreases bitterness in olive oil and US consumers actually prefer the taste of rancid oil[118]. The US is known as "the world's dumping ground for rancid and defective olive oil" says Sue Langstaff, a sensory scientist and author of Olive Oil Sensory Science[119]. A 2010 report by UC Davis found 69% of olive oils imported into the US and 10% of California grown oils did not meet International Olive Council standards because they were either rancid, adulterated or contained off flavors from fruit fly infestation, delayed processing etc[120].

Here is what you can do to reduce the likelihood of eating rancid fats in the diet while on the trail.
1. Purchase the freshest fats. The fresher the better, any unsaturated fat older than 1 year old has a very high chance of being rancid. Buy only olive oil from the most recent harvest, it must have a date stamp less than a year old and be from California.
2. Purchase fats that are kept in cool, low light settings such as the oil in the back of the shelf away from light.
3. Store fats in cool dark environments, away from the stove, heater or window at home. Ask the person who is shipping your food to keep meals high in unsaturated fats in their fridge until shipping (i.e. peanut oil cream, soups with vegetable oil). On the trail, keep your food in the relatively cool center of your pack, this includes fish oil capsules.

4. Don't mail drop food more than one month ahead, sitting in a hot post office will increase rancidification.
5. Use airtight containers and reseal the cap immediately after use. If transporting oil in a Nalgene bag, purge as much air as possible before closing.
6. Vacuum seal foods. This is especially important for meat and fat combinations such as pemmican as the iron in the meat speeds up oxidative rancidification[121].
7. Render fats thoroughly. Rendered fats such as tallow, lard and ghee are fats that have been heated at low temperatures to evaporate all the water to prevent hydrolytic and microbial rancidification (without water, very few microbes can survive).
8. Be extra careful with unsaturated fats. The more unsaturated a fat is, the more at risk it is to oxidative rancidification because each additional carbon that is missing a hydrogen atom is a potential site for oxidation. Rendered saturated fats and coconut oil are at lowest risk of oxidative rancidification, followed by oils high in monounsaturated fats such as olive, avocado oil and high-oleic sunflower and safflower oil. The fats at greatest risk of oxidative rancidification are vegetable oils and these should not be mail dropped more than a few weeks ahead. These include peanut, canola, sesame, cottonseed, sunflower, soybean, safflower and flaxseed oil.
9. Avoid any baked or preserved foods that contain omega-3 as this oil is highly susceptible to oxidative rancidification and will almost certainly be rancid.
10.
onsume antioxidant rich foods with high fat meals.

Rancidification cannot be completely avoided as the stomach and intestines are a warm place full of enzymes that break down fat and the mere act of digestion involves some oxidative rancidification[122].

When consumed in the same meal, the antioxidants present in fresh leafy greens have been shown to neutralize and reduce the absorption of oxidative rancidification byproducts such as free radicals[123]. This is already difficult to do on the trail as fresh vegetables are not available other than what can be foraged and even more difficult on a ketogenic diet given the fact that many antioxidant rich foods contain too many carbohydrates to maintain ketosis.

Several recipes in this book contain antioxidant rich fruit powders and antioxidant supplements can be easily found. Some antioxidant intake is good, but there is an upper limit as excessive anti-oxidant intake can have cancer promoting effects[3,124].

There is theoretical evidence that fat metabolism produces fewer dangerous free radicals than the metabolism of carbohydrates[2]. It is hard to tell where the ketogenic backpacking diet falls on the spectrum of net oxidative damage from fat digestion and metabolism when compared to other common backpacking diets. In any case, it is prudent to take precautions against consuming rancid oil, as a diet is only as healthy as the ingredients it is composed of.

7. A Guide to Healthy Proteins

To maintain a state of nutritional ketosis, your protein intake must be moderate. But does the type of protein matter? There are three things worth mentioning about protein type within the context of a ketogenic diet while backpacking.

1. Complete proteins and vegetarianism
2. Other components of protein rich foods
3. Biological activity of proteins

Most of the structure of your body is made up of protein, this includes your organs, blood vessels and most of your connective tissue including skin, fascia and muscle. These structures are constantly being repaired and replaced at an astounding rate. The lining of your small intestine is completely replaced every 4 days, skin every 30 days and muscle every 5 months[125]. This means that by the time you have completed a thru hike, you are hiking with new guts, skin and legs. While some of the proteins comprising these structures are recycled, much of it must come from the diet. If you are made of the protein you eat, does it matter what type of protein you eat?

When it comes to the protein itself, the surprising answer is, not really, as long as all the amino acids are present. Proteins are made up of molecular building blocks called amino acids and the amino acid lysine is the same whether it was derived from a pork chop or an almond.

Vegetarians and Vegans

Your body is capable of interconverting many of these amino acids but there are nine amino acids that it cannot interconvert and must obtain from the diet. These are called essential amino acids.

Animal proteins will contain all nine essential amino acids and are thus considered complete.

Lacto-ovo vegetarians eat eggs and fish which are both sources of all nine essential amino acids. Lacto-ovo vegetarians will have no difficulty getting complete proteins on a ketogenic diet if they make these foods their primary protein sources.

However, a single plant source of protein will have some combination of essential amino acids but not all of them. For example, legumes such as peanuts have plenty of the essential amino acid lysine but are lacking in methionine, while grains such as wheat have plenty of methionine while lacking lysine. The combination of a peanut butter sandwich results in a complete protein. This occurs effortlessly when eating a combination of different plant sources and there is no need to carefully match complementary proteins at each meal[126]. But what if you are on the ketogenic diet and eat peanut butter with butter and no bread? The answer is: you are still lacking in methionine and must find another source for it.

If you are eating a limited vegetarian or vegan ketogenic diet while backpacking, you will find it challenging to get all nine amino acids due to the combination of a moderate protein intake and the lack of animal proteins. In this situation, I recommend planning meals carefully to ensure complete protein intake and relying heavily on a complete protein source such as a vegan protein powder. You can use a food database such as https://chronometer.com to calculate the essential amino acid content of your backpacking menu.

Other Components of Protein-Rich Foods

As far as muscle building and tissue repair is concerned, if you are getting all the essential amino acids, it doesn't matter where they come from. But this doesn't mean that an ounce of blue cheese and an ounce of wild caught sardines will have the same overall effects on your body. Protein rich foods rarely contain only protein. There are many other compounds present in protein rich foods besides the protein that influence health. These include 1) the type of fats 2) vitamins and minerals 3) biological activity of the unique protein structure itself and 4) toxins, additives and compounds.

Fats found in protein rich foods
Grass fed sources of animal protein will contain more anti-inflammatory omega-3 fats and less pro-inflammatory omega-6 fats than their grain fed counterparts[127]. Wild caught, cold water fish have the most healthy omega-3 fat of any source.

Vitamins and minerals in protein rich foods
organ meats are the vegetables of a carnivore's diet. The artic Inuit traditionally lived exclusively on raw and lightly cooked meat, blubber and organs for many months out of the year without any apparent nutrient deficiencies[128]. Meat eaten raw within hours of slaughter will even retain vitamin C and liver, pancreas, and thyroid glands are packed with vitamins and minerals. For example, a 3.5 ounce (100g) serving of liver contains 7,744mcg of vitamin A, nearly 10x as much as you would synthesize from eating the same weight of carrots (835mcg)[129,130]. However, it is unlikely that you will be subsisting on raw or lightly cooked freshly killed wild game on your backpacking trip and the preserved animal products available to you have nutrient imbalances that are important to compensate for. See the following chapter on vitamins and minerals for more details.

Biologically Active Proteins

Many of the hormones your body uses to send signals between different regions are made of protein. Thus, if a protein you eat makes it through the digestion and into the bloodstream without being fully dismantled it is possible for it to have a hormonal effect.

The most notable and disputable food in this category is dairy. Cheese and butter are very convenient and delicious foods for ketogenic backpacking. Dairy products have measurable levels of hormones with plausible biological action in humans[131]. However large scale epidemiological studies have found only a few reliable results, namely that men who consume the most whole milk have the highest rates of prostate cancer while women with the highest consumption of high fat dairy were the least likely to become overweight or obese[132-134]. It seems that dairy intake will have different effects on different people, I recommend testing dairy products out on yourself so see how you respond.

Of note, lactose intolerance is of little consequence on a ketogenic diet, as the dairy products that are ketogenic (hard cheese and butter) are extremely low in the milk sugar lactose.

Proteins are also used by the immune system to identify intruders and some proteins can activate the immune system and cause either a local inflammatory response in the digestive tract or a more systemic allergic response. Allergies are person-specific, and one person may eat peanuts with impunity while another can literally die from eating almond butter out of a jar that contained peanut butter. Despite the idiosyncrasies of the immune system, there seem to be some foods that are more likely to provoke an immune response. The majority of food allergies are diagnosed in childhood or adolescence but 15% are diagnosed in adulthood[135]. Here is a list of those foods, if you have suspicions about your response to any of these foods (i.e. had stomach upset or hives after eating one of these foods) I recommend excluding it from your backcountry menu planning and or carrying an EpiPen as an allergic response when far from medical care is a serious problem.

List of foods people are often allergic to[135].
- Milk
- Eggs
- Peanuts
- Tree Nuts
- Soy
- Sesame
- Wheat
- Fish
- Shellfish

Browning
The Maillard reaction is a form of non-enzymatic browning that produces the delicious flavors and aromas of browned meat, onions etc. Unfortunately, at higher temperatures, the Maillard reactions produce a potential carcinogen called acrylamide as well as other heterocyclic aromatic amines and polycyclic aromatic hydrocarbons. These mutagens may be responsible for the fact that people who regularly ate heavily browned meat had 6.0x higher rectal cancer and 2.8x higher colon cancer rates[136]. Not all studies have found this association between darkly browned meats and cancer, but there is sufficient evidence to give you pause before frying your salami every night[137,138].

Processed Meats
Speaking of salami, if the saturated fat and cholesterol content are not a problem, what about the processing itself? Does eating processed meat increase the risk of cancer? The epidemiological research suggests this to be the case as the relative risk of colorectal cancer increased by 24% for

each additional 120g of red meat and by 36% for each additional 30g of processed meat consumed each day[139]. However, it is not clear how much of this effect is due to the high omega-6 content of the meats being consumed in these studies versus the processing itself. Cancer rates have been reportedly low among hunter gathers eating a diet high in omega-3 rich wild game , including the artic Inuit who obtain >90% of their calories from animal products during most of the year[140]fish.

Mercury in Fish

Mercury is a neurotoxin that is released into the air by coal burning power plants, smelting and waste incineration and enters the water where it is consumed by wildlife[141]. The higher a species is on the food chain the more mercury it will accumulate. The highest levels of mercury are found in apex predators such as sharks, seals, swordfish, king mackerel and tuna but mercury is so toxic and so prevalent in the environment that the levels found in most fish are potentially dangerous, especially if eaten daily. Mercury's damaging effects on the nervous system are a cause of concern for everyone but those whose brains are developing experience the greatest harm[142]. Blood mercury levels have begun to decrease as people choose to eat lower mercury fish but as of 2010, 1 in 6 women of childbearing age in coastal areas of the US had levels high enough to impair child development[143].

Polychlorinated Biphenyl in Farmed Fish

Farmed fish is fed grain containing cancer causing pesticides such as polychlorinated biphenyls (PCBs) which are concentrated in the fish bodies[144]. Furthermore, grain-fed fish have which results in high omega-6 and low

53

omega-3 fatty acids just like grain fed land animals. Not only does farmed fish lack most of the health benefits of wild caught fish, fish farming is also done in a way that negatively impacts the environment.

The healthiest seafood is both high in omega-3 and low in toxins such as mercury and PCB's. This includes wild caught:

- Sardines
- Mackerel
- Anchovies
- Salmon
- Herring

Use the acronym S.M.A.S.H to remember these healthy fish.

Other seafood that is safe but does not contain as much omega-3 includes:
- Butterfish
- Crab (domestic)
- Crawfish
- Clam
- Croaker (Atlantic)
- Mullet
- Perch (Ocean)
- Plaice
- Pollock
- Shad (American)
- Sole (Pacific)
- Squid
- Tilapia
- Trout (freshwater)

8. Micronutrients

Whole foods are your best source of vitamins and minerals, and among these whole foods the most concentrated sources are fresh vegetables and organ meats both of which are difficult to get while backpacking. Wild foraged plants often have 10x more vitamins and minerals than agricultural vegetables but searching for them and consuming them requires some expertise, time and a tolerance for bitter flavors. This is a worthwhile project if you are doing 8 miles a day, but is extremely difficult when you are trying to cover 20+ as it often involves going off trail.

A ketogenic diet consisting of the recipes in this book will easily supply all the fat-soluble vitamins: A, D, E and K. However, you will likely need a supplement containing the water-soluble vitamins found in fresh vegetables (vitamin C and all the B vitamins). It is important that this supplement contain relatively low levels of fat-soluble vitamins A, D, E and K as these can accumulate in your body to toxic levels with over-supplementation.

The combination of a ketogenic diet and backpacking all day warrant paying some attention to the intake of two key minerals: sodium and potassium.

Sodium

Sodium is a mineral that is critically involved in basic cell functions, but the body has no sodium storage, so it must be consumed frequently to maintain adequate levels.

Sodium levels are very low in most plant foods so people living far from the ocean had to made great efforts to obtain enough sodium[145]. For example, the Gidra-speaking Papuans of the Orimo Plateau would burn Melaleuca trees and consume the bitter ash to obtain small amounts of sodium[146]. Other groups would trade valuable goods for salt or walk long distances to obtain it. The scarcity of salt combined with its importance likely explains why we find it so delicious.

In the modern world, salt is plentiful and because it is a food preservative, backpackers will typically have more than enough salt in their diet. This is typically true of a ketogenic backpacking diet as salami, cheese, salted nut butters, salmon skin chips, seaweed, dried fish, broth and soup mixes are all loaded with sodium.

Even so, you are more likely to have a sodium deficiency on a ketogenic diet because the chronically low insulin levels result in low levels of anti-diuretic hormone (ADH)[2]. ADH is the hormone responsible for sodium retention and when ADH is low you excrete more salt in your urine. This salt loss in your urine combined with salt loss from sweat on a long hiking day in high heat and humidity could leave you low on sodium if you are not consuming any sodium-rich foods or beverages.

In addition to basic cellular functions, sodium is responsible for maintaining blood volume. Low sodium is called hyponatremia and results in cellular swelling with symptoms that can include any or all the following: fainting, nausea, headache, confusion and fatigue[147]. Furthermore, when sodium levels are low, the kidneys will begin to excrete potassium to maintain sodium levels which can result in low potassium[2].

Risk factors for hyponatremia include exercising for more than 3 hours, excessive sweating, diarrhea and drinking too much water without ingesting any sodium[147]. These are all things hikers are likely to face.

The solution is simple: aim for at least 3,000mg of sodium per day, with intake spread throughout the day[2].

This is easily accomplished by having broth for breakfast, salted nut butter or seaweed for lunch and a salty soup for dinner. Larger athletes hiking farther and faster on hotter and more humid days will need considerably more.

Is this too much sodium? The Centers for Disease Control reports that the average American consumes 3,400mg of sodium per day and recommends restricting this to 2,300mg[148]. The CDC states this guideline is primarily out of a concern for a high sodium intake increasing your blood pressure although this effect of sodium is only seen in a subset of sodium-sensitive people who already have high blood pressure[149,150]. On a ketogenic diet this sodium is more rapidly excreted and thus unlikely to elevated blood pressure[2]. Independently of blood pressure, both very low (<2,645mg) and very high (>4,945mg) sodium intakes are associated with death of all causes[151].

If you are concerned about your blood pressure on the ketogenic diet, measure it for one week on your typical diet and record your sodium intake, then measure for a week on the ketogenic diet as described in this book with 3,000mg of sodium per day. Be sure to measure in the same position at rest and compare the results. For individuals over the age of 65, African Americans or those with a diagnosis of hypertension, it would be prudent to calibrate your salt intake before setting off on your hike by consulting with your physician and monitoring your blood pressure[148].

Potassium

Another potential electrolyte experienced by backpackers is too little potassium.
Potassium is lost in sweat and feces but not found as plentifully in processed foods as sodium is. Low potassium

is called hypokalemia and can cause weakness, cramping, numbness, tingling, nausea, abdominal bloating and cramping, constipation and heart palpitations. Risk factors for hypokalemia are the same as for hyponatremia including excessive sweating, diarrhea and drinking too much water without ingesting any sodium or potassium.

If the short term, deficiency of either of these minerals can have serious and immediate consequences that can take you off the trail. But in the long run, the balance of these minerals is important. Specifically, a diet high in sodium and low in potassium has been consistently linked to heart disease[152].

Inadequate potassium is especially likely for those on a ketogenic diet as the foods highest in potassium are also high in carbs: potatoes, tomatoes, beans and dried fruit. Dark leafy greens are also high in potassium and any foraged along the trail will be helpful.

Fish and bone broths are the best sources of potassium for the ketogenic backpacker but since current food labels are not required to state the amount of potassium, ensuring adequate intake from prepared foods is difficult. Supplementing with potassium is possible but should be done with caution and always taken with water. Healthy kidneys can easily shed a little extra potassium, but damaged kidneys, dehydration or excessively high potassium intake carries the risk of blood potassium levels risking too high, a state called hyperkalemia. The risks of high potassium are more acute than high sodium levels, namely heart palpitations, chest pain and difficulty breathing in addition to fatigue, nausea, vomiting, numbness and tingling. If you have kidney dysfunction, check with your doctor before supplementing with potassium.

The safest and most reliable way to maintain adequate and balanced sodium and potassium levels while hiking on a ketogenic diet is to regularly consume a sugar free electrolyte supplement. On less strenuous or cooler day, this can be done as little as once a day, however in high heat and humidity put electrolytes in all the water you drink.

9. Gastro-intestinal Health

A diet that is 90% fat can present several digestive challenges that require consideration. People vary greatly in their digestive function and you may find that eating a ketogenic diet improves your digestion, or you may find it very challenging[2][153][154]. I was unable to find much research specifically investigating the effects of a ketogenic diet on gastro-intestinal function and thus much of the following chapter is based on a combination of anecdotes from myself and others as well as inferences made from studies of basic digestive physiology. Use this information as a starting point, and experiment to find what works for you.

I believe that the more of the following characteristics you have, the more likely you will be to have difficulty with gastro-intestinal adaption to the ketogenic diet: 1) previously ate a low-fat diet, 2) have had you're your gall bladder removed (cholecystectomy) 3) frequent suffer from constipation, 4) need to eat a lot of calories.

Poor gastro-intestinal tolerance of the ketogenic diet generally takes one of two forms:
1. **Inadequate absorption**. If fats pass through the small intestine undigested, they will either be digested by the bacteria of the large intestine which produce gas that stretches the intestine causing bloating and pain or they will pass all the way through undigested causing an oily stool. The first is uncomfortable, the latter is wasteful at best and "disaster pants" at worst.
2. **Constipation.** Fats are generally completely digested and leave little behind to bulk up the stool. Fiber speeds up gastric motility and both bulks and softens stool

---

[2] Some studies show increasing fat intake speeds up gastric emptying and intestinal transit time and others show no difference. The effect likely varies by type of fat and personal factors.

making it easier to pass. The combination of a high fat and low fiber intake together increases the risk of constipation[44]. At best this means several days go by without visiting a privy or touching your stash of TP. At worst it means an agonizing internment in a privy prison complete with horrific odors, cobwebs and someone knocking on the door.

Fortunately, these challenges are relatively easily overcome with a basic understanding of fat digestion, and a few dietary adjustments to suite your system.

Fat Digestion Basics

To digest fat, you must 1) break it down into small pieces, 2) make it water soluble, and 3) absorb it into your blood stream.

First, you must break fat down into small enough pieces to pass through the intestinal lining. Most dietary fat comes in the form of triglycerides that must be broken down into free fatty acids and monoglycerides. This begins in your mouth with an enzyme called oral lipase and continues in your stomach with gastric lipase and in your small intestine and stomach with pancreatic lipase.

Second, you must make the fat water soluble by binding it to an emulsifier such as those released into your small intestine by the gall bladder and liver[155]. This process of making fats water soluble is called emulsification.

As your oral and gastric lipase breaks triglycerides down into fatty acids, these fatty acids stimulate the release of cholecystokinin from the wall of the small intestine. Cholecystokinin, abbreviated CCK, contributes to your feeling of fullness and signals the release of bile from the gall bladder. Bile is made by your liver but stored in the gall bladder to allow a large amount to be release all at once. Even so, a typical moderately fatty meal will require more bile than your gall bladder can store. Fortunately, bile is reabsorbed from the intestinal wall after it is used and sent back to the liver. Your liver also continues to produce and secrete bile during a meal to accommodate for a larger quantity of fat.

Third, fats must enter your blood stream and they do this through either the intestinal blood vessels or special lymphatic ducts called lacteals.

Short and medium chain fatty acids are found most plentifully in coconut oil and butter and are small enough to be absorbed directly into the intestinal blood stream and sent to the liver where they are either used as fuel for the liver, or converted to ketones and sent on to the rest of the blood stream[156].

Most fats consist primarily of long chain fatty acids. They are too long to be absorbed directly into the intestinal bloodstream and must bypass the liver and take a special lymphatic route into your bloodstream[44]. First, they enter the cells of the small intestine where they are recombined to form triglycerides and then connected to phospholipids to keep them water soluble in a structure called a chylomicron. These chylomicrons form a milky substance called chyle which is transported by your lymphatics ducts (lacteals) from your small intestine up to the left subclavian vein just below your left collar bone where they enter your bloodstream. Long chain triglycerides begin to show up in the bloodstream 2 hours after a meal, peak at 5 hours and are generally cleared by 10 hours[44]. Once in your the bloodstream, the fatty acids in the chylomicrons are slowly picked apart by lipoprotein lipase in the heart, muscle and fat cells to be burned or stored according to energy demands.

Solutions for Poor Absorption

With this understanding of fat digestion, lets discuss some solutions to the problem of poor fat absorption.

1. **Start Slow**
   From your current diet, gradual replace carbohydrates and protein in your meals until you reach a Wilder ratio of 4 grams of fat for every combined 1 gram of carbohydrates and protein. Reaching a full ketogenic diet may take several weeks if you have been eating a low-fat diet but this allows your body time to increase bile and lipase production.

2. **Eat Slowly and Calmly**
   Eat slowly and calmly to give your body plenty of time to release bile and lipase. Avoid eating when stressed as the stress response decreases gastric acid secretion, reduces blood flow to the stomach, inhibits intestinal motility and reduces food propulsion[157]. Some of the recipes in this book are dangerously delicious and require very little chewing. It is easy to eat a whole cup of spicy Thai cashew cream in a matter of minutes, overwhelm your bile and lipase secretion rates and suffer poor absorption, but the same dose spread out over an hour could be digested without issue. If you are doing big miles and need to eat a lot of calories, try eating 4-5 smaller meals instead of 3 larger meals.

3. **Pre-Emulsify**
   Fats are not water soluble, but the human body is mostly water. If you consume more fat at a time than

your gall bladder has bile to emulsify, fat passes through undigested. One solution is to emulsify the fat before consuming it[158]. Many of the recipes in this book call for the use of soy lecithin with this goal in mind. If you are having trouble digesting a recipe, try doubling the amount of lecithin in a recipe or adding lecithin to any meal you seem to be having trouble digesting.

4. Supplement with digestive enzymes.
A variety of supplements are available to help your digestive system out with the process of breaking down and emulsifying fats. These supplements are usually necessary if your gall bladder has been removed (cholecystectomy) and recommended if you need to eat a lot of calories. As with any case where you are supplementing something that your body produces naturally, I recommend using the minimum dose necessary and gradually weaning off the supplement as able to prevent your body from down-regulating its own production.

Lipase
Lipase breaks down fats into smaller pieces and can be taken as a supplement in capsule form. Take these with meals and balance the dose as needed to ensure digestion. The dose will vary according to the amount of fat in the meal, how fast you eat and how much lipase your body produces naturally.

Bile
If you aren't making enough of your own bile, you can eat someone else's. This may sound off-putting but these days, ox bile comes in capsules to make the process easier. Purchase the smaller dose capsule (125mg) and take one capsule with meals. Increase the dose at subsequent meals until you achieve the desired effect, but beware, too high of a dose will overload the

enterohepatic circulation's ability to recycle the bile and it will end up in your stool causing a burning sensation upon exit. Freeze dried liver also contains a small amount of bile in addition to many vitamins and minerals and may be a better tolerated source.

5. **Identify Trigger foods**
   Some foods will cause an inflammatory or mild allergic reaction in the small intestine that will impair absorption. Suspect foods include nuts, shellfish, tomatoes, garlic, onion, spicy and acidic food. Record which meals result in digestive symptoms, remove the suspect ingredient and try again. Often it is not the oil that is the irritant but rather the protein. I can consume 1,000kcal of peanut oil set with glycerides but would suffer diarrhea from the same number of calories in the form of peanut butter.

6. **Change your MCT oil intake.**
   Medium chain triglycerides are touted as brain fuel because of their quick digestibility and easy conversion to ketones. However, they are also well known to cause digestive upset. The simplest way to avoid this issue is to avoid MCTs either in pure form or fats that contain high quantities of MCT, namely coconut oil. But this also means missing out on the potential benefits of MCTs.

   Why is MCT oil so prone to cause abdominal pain, bloating, gas and diarrhea?
   There are several reasons for this problem, a few are inherent to MCT and the rest are avoidable.

   Inherent Challenges with MCT Oil

   1. **Antimicrobial effects.**

As a group, medium chain triglycerides have powerful antimicrobial effects which means they kill bacteria and fungus[159-161]. This is especially true of C8 (Caprylic acid)[162,163]. Theoretically this is a good thing as most of this effect should be occurring in the stomach and small intestine, two areas that should be kept relatively clear of microbes. However, when microbes are split open by MCT, the resulting pieces activate an inflammatory reaction in the intestine that brings water into the intestine causing diarrhea. This effect is greatly magnified if some MCT makes it farther down into the microbe-rich large intestine where the resulting carnage leaves a trail of debris and disrupts the healthy microbial balance.

2. MCT Absorption Rate

The medium chain triglycerides C8 (Caprylic acid) and C10 (Capric acid) require lipase to be broken down into fatty acids and glycerol but then can pass through the intestinal lining and into the blood stream directly without the need for bile[156]. If the amount of MCT consumed overwhelms the available lipase, trouble ensues.

One way around these challenges is to dose your MCT judiciously. Like other dietary fats, smaller doses spread out throughout the day are better tolerated. I recommend starting with 1tsp with a meal and if tolerated, adding another teaspoon later in the day. Even those who tolerate MCT well usually top out at 3 tablespoons (14g) spread out throughout the day. Even so, extremely high doses of MCT oil have been used to control seizures, with one author reporting use of a diet comprising up to 40-70% of calories from MCT oil[81] Patients are admitted to the hospital for their adaptation period. Their meals start at 1/3 of normal size and if they experience vomiting or diarrhea they are given anti-nausea suppositories and IV fluids while not being allowed to drink[81]. Apparently, most patients adapt to the high MCT intake and continue the diet after leaving the hospital[81]. I find this astounding given my own experience of gastrointestinal distress at a mere 8% of calories from MCT oil.

Supplementation with lipase is another option since MCT digestion depends on lipase. But bile supplementation is unlikely to be helpful.

A third option is to switch from liquid MCT oil to MCT oil powder. To make powdered MCT oil, liquid MCT oil is sprayed through a fine powder such as soluble corn fiber to produce a powdered oil that is much easier to transport and dissolve than liquid oil. Anecdotally many people report being able to take a higher dose of MCT oil powder than liquid MCT oil without gastrointestinal symptoms and this has certainly been the case for me.

Avoidable Challenges with MCT Oil

There are a few reasons MCT oil might be causing poor absorption that depend primarily on the type of MCT oil you are consuming. MCT oil advocate Dave Asprey, author of the Bulletproof Diet and Head Strong, claims solvents and lauric acid present in MCT oil can both cause gastrointestinal upset[8,164]. I was unable to find any scientific research addressing this topic specifically, but I recommend purchasing different oils and testing them out on yourself.

Cheap MCT oil is often a byproduct of the cosmetic industry which was extracted using solvents. This MCT oil may contain the solvent hexanes which is an intestinal irritation, C17 which is a byproduct of solvent extraction or C6 which is a poorly digested MCT that would otherwise be removed.

Lauric acid (C12) is technically a medium chain triglyceride but is too long to be absorbed directly into the bloodstream the way C8 (caprylic acid) and C10 (capric acid) are and must go through the process of long chain triglyceride digestion involving lipase and bile. Although C12 has many health benefits, its requirements for bile and lipase in addition to its antimicrobial properties make it likely culprit in digestive upset at high doses.

One solution to these problems is to consume a higher quality oil that is extracted by expeller pressing without solvents and/or consume pure C8 oil (caprylic acid) to see if you tolerate it better.

Solutions for Constipation

If your fiber intake is low, the solution to constipation is the same whether or not you are on a ketogenic diet: drink sufficient water and eat more fiber. A systematic review of the scientific research on the topic found that increasing fiber intake reduced constipation in 77% of subjects[165,166]. In food this would take the form of eating more nuts and seeds as well as high fiber, low carbohydrate leafy greens foraged along the trail such dandelion and plantain. A much more expedient method is to take a daily fiber supplement containing insoluble fiber as this is the type of fiber that speeds transit time and brings water into the stool. This could consist of any number of fiber sources including wheat bran, inulin, methylcellulose and psyllium. Start off with a moderate dose with each meal and increase until you achieve the desired result.

Constipation may also be caused by medications such as opiate pain medication, antidepressants, antipsychotics and some antacids as well as irritable bowel and inflammatory bowel syndromes. People vary greatly in their digestive function, and in some people decreasing fiber improves constipation[167].

Laxatives such as milk of magnesia can be used in a pinch, but the regular use of these may impair nutrient absorption. Carrying all that food out into the woods and then not being able to fully digest it may be a great way to lose weight but it's neither healthy or enjoyable.

In summary, whether the ketogenic diet is digestive smooth sailing or rough water depends on your own digestive characteristics and the number of calories you need to consume. The massive caloric intake required by some speed hikers always presents digestive challenges and when compared to the digestive challenges many others face on the trail from their undercooked freeze-dried food and binging in trail towns the ketogenic diet looks quite manageable.

III: PREPARING THE KETOGENIC DIET

10. Menu Planning

Why Variety Matters

The ketogenic diet is a clear winner for the ultralight backpacker. The smug satisfaction of carrying half the weight for the same number of calories and feeling energized is enough for some to eat only butter and cheese all day. If this is you, go ahead and skip this chapter and plan your menu making sure you have enough variety to get all your nutrients. But if you are someone for whom food is more than a utilitarian calculation of calories and nutrition, someone who wants to enjoy and look forward to your meals, this chapter is for you.

For thru hikers, with long days on the trail, the pleasure of food often becomes a fixation. The ketogenic diet can be deeply satisfying, (nothing like bacon after a long hike) but susceptible to boredom on the trail because so many standard hiking foods are excluded, and the lack of refrigeration makes many standard ketogenic meals impossible (so much for fresh bacon). Indeed, it is this very reason that I wrote this cookbook.

In addition to keeping a menu interesting, a varied menu is healthier because it is less likely to have too much or too little of any given nutrient.

How to Create Variety

To remain interesting, meals must vary in both taste and texture. A diverse menu of savory dishes will likely still become boring without a few sweeter foods mixed in. Because of its high fat content, the ketogenic diet naturally tends towards soft and creamy textures, so be sure to balance these with meals that have chewy and crunchy textures.

How Much Variety?

A simple diet simplifies packing. If you planned to eat the same thing for every meal, packing your hiker boxes for six months would be a breeze… but eating them would be a chore. Conversely, trying to have a different meal each day is easy to do for a weekend trip but becomes a logistical nightmare for a thru hike. The ideal amount of variety lies somewhere in the middle.

I recommend taking a survey of the variety in your meals over the last few weeks and aim for a similar variety, erring slightly on the side of more variety. My wife and I like to pack three different breakfasts, lunches, snacks and dinners for a six-day resupply, with each meal repeating once. Then for the next weeks box we would change out a few of the meals.

One major consideration for meal variety is efficiency of ingredient use. The size of the packages your ingredients come in determine how many batches you can make of a recipe without any leftovers. When packing for a thru hike it can be frustrating and expensive to have a little bit of this and that left over in different jars. For this reason, I have written many of the recipes to have serving sizes that evenly divide the standard containers of the larger and more expensive ingredients.

How Many Calories?

Calculating the appropriate number of calories to bring on a backpacking trip is a difficult task. Caloric expenditure varies greatly between individuals and by hiking terrain. I recommend starting by using the metabolic equivalent tables to estimate your hiking expenditure and adding this on top of your estimate resting metabolic rate[168]. Bring a little extra and go for a weekend or better yet a week long backpacking trip and see how much you eat. If you are trying to lose weight, bring a little less food, but I caution you against severely under-packing food because it increases the chance that you will be very hungry and end up eating foods that will suppress fat burning.

11. Storing and Packing

Packing by Meal vs by Ingredient
While we were packing our resupply boxes for two months on the Appalachian trail, my wife and I faced the question of whether to pack by meal or by ingredient.

Packing by meal involves measuring out the exact quantities for each meal individually and packing them together as a stand-alone meal. Essentially doing everything but cooking it ahead of time. I compare this to making and bringing MREs. It is tedious and time consuming to measure out all the ingredients for each meal in advance, but the advantage was that once all the ingredients of a meal are packed together, it was easy to make changes in the menu.

Packing by ingredient involves packing enough of each ingredient for several meals separately and then do both the mixing and the heating on the trail. This is a lot more like bringing your pantry with you on the trail. It's a lot faster to pack up at home, but it gets very complex if you are trying to eat a diverse menu and can become a Gordian knot when trying to make menu changes.
We ended up packing mostly by individual meal for our first Appalachian trail section hike. For our next section we will pack breakfast and dinner by ingredient as these tend to have a large amount of liquid oil that is best kept in its own Nalgene bag and pack lunch by meal to allow for more variety.

Managing Oils
Managing oils on the trail can be a mess. For our 700-mile Appalachian Trail section hike we heat-sealed most of our dinners in Mylar bags. A few of these bags leaked either through the seal or through puncture and coated the rest of

the food in our food bag resulting in all our food tasting like olive oil, and costing us many frustrating minutes of licking oily fingers in a world where you can't just grab a paper towel and wipe things up. More than once I have thrown a stick of butter or a few chunks of coconut oil into a plastic bag forgetting that mid-afternoon the oil will have melted and leaked all over my pack. Take my advice and pack your oils securely even if it means using heavier containers. Here are my recommendations for packing oils or anything that may leak.

Plastic containers
Tightly sealing plastic Tupperware such as those made by Lock & Lock brand are durable and safe. They are too heavy for most thru hikers, but you may find them worth the weight for shorter trips. Reused plastic nut butter jars are lighter and seal nearly as well. One empty Trader Joe's raw almond butter jar weighs 1.5oz (43 grams).

Bags
Plastic bags make for ultralight storage, but you don't see people hiking with Ziploc bags of water and for the same reason I don't recommend packing anything ketogenic in Ziploc bags. Instead, for large quantities, the tightly sealing Nalgene wide mouth canteen bag is a good option. The 32oz bag weighs 2.1oz (59g). I haven't seen a smaller size, and it would probably not be as efficient because most of the weight is in the large cap. Carrying such a large amount of one ingredient is weight efficient and simplifies meal prep but reduces variety. Mild flavored oils such as avocado or strained coconut oil are best for bagging because they can be used in many recipes.

Fitting it All in a Bear Canister
To protect your food and keep wildlife wild, it is necessary to carry your food in a bear canister. Some parks in the US such as Great Smokey Mountains National Park, and

Yosemite National Park require these wildlife-proof containers for all backcountry camping. While these bear canisters are good for the environment, they present some challenges in packing as they are heavy and provide limited space. When packing in a bear canister I recommend bagging all dry ingredients, and packing liquid ingredients in Nalgene wide mouth canteen bags to allow the items to conform to the limited space.

12. Cooking on the Trail

Cooking the recipes in the book requires nothing more than heating water and mixing ingredients. I recommend using a lightweight butane stove such as the JetBoil Firelite exclusively for heating water and then mixing your meals in a Nalgene bottle or bowl. This prevents the problem of burning food in the stove pot and the subsequent headache of cleaning it on the trail. I licked my bowls and rinsed my bottles immediately and saved weight by not bringing any dish cleaning supplies.

13. Creating New Recipes

New Recipe Templates

In this section, I hope to inspire you to go "off-trail" and come up with your own ketogenic backpacking recipes. With a little guidance and the help of the two formulas below you can create delicious meals perfectly suited to your own needs and preferences.

Here is a formula for creating a ketogenic backpacking meal I call the "Ketogenic Replica"

1. Identify a favorite meal
2. Identify the primary sources of fat and quadruple the amount
3. Exchange carbohydrates with low carb sources that are similar in texture.
4. Find backpacking friendly versions of all remaining ingredients.
5. Make the first batch with a Wilder ratio of 4:1 (grams of fat/ carbs + protein).
6. Adjust the ingredient ratios based on the above result to balance goals of flavor and fueling.

Here is another formula for creating a ketogenic meal I call "Bootstrapping:

1. Identify a fat source you like.
2. Brainstorm taste parings in each of the following three categories:
   a. hot beverage
   b. soup
   c. cream/dip.
3. Add ingredients that provide textural variety.

4. Make the first batch with a Wilder ratio of 4:1 (grams of fat/ carbs + protein).
5. Adjust the ingredient ratios based on the above result to balance goals of flavor and fueling.

Salting

Salt has a multitude of benefits for the backpacker. First, salt is a vital electrolyte that must be replaced after sweating. Second, salt increases the shelf life of food. Third, salt improves the flavor of food by reducing the perception of bitterness and enhancing other previously overlooked tastes. Salt even increases the perception of sweetness.

When improvising ketogenic backpacking recipes, one should be aware that salt does not dissolve in fat. This is particularly relevant for water-free dishes such as pemmican, nut butters and dips. The solution is to add salt to the recipe via pre-salted ingredients instead of pouring salt in directly. For example, to adjust the saltiness of a butter and nut butter blend, use either salted or unsalted butter and salted or unsalted nut butter. This adjustment of salt in a dish through the conscious use of salty ingredients is called "salt layering" by chef and food writer Samin Nosrat, and is a useful tool for the ketogenic backpacking cook[169].

Non-caloric Sweeteners

A review of the research on non-caloric sweeteners found they have little impact on insulin and appetite. Still, if you are struggling to lose weight, it's worth testing their effects on you[170].

Stevia is the least processed of the non-caloric sweeteners because it is extracted from the leaves of Stevia rebaudiana plant. Even so, stevia has about 60% of the insulin stimulating effect as table sugar, certainly an improvement, but consuming large and frequent quantities of stevia will result in an insulin response than will reduce fat metabolism[171]. Also, stevia is metabolized by gut bacteria into a substance called steviol which is both cancer causing or cancer killing in laboratory tests[172,173]. Most artificial sweeteners on the market have been proven safe in studies of several months duration, although the impact of high levels of consumption over a lifetime is unknown.

If on the other hand, you fear your appetite is not keeping up with what you are burning, you may consider sweetening things up a little bit. Sweetness aside, people eat more when given a variety of foods and less when given less variety, regardless of the types of food[174]. Having delicious and interesting food can stimulate you to eat primarily for the pleasure of eating, and this "eating for entertainment" is not calibrated to your caloric need. Theoretically this is less of an issue on a ketogenic diet because of the key role carbohydrates, and sugar, play in the hijacking of appetite by the reward center of the brain but I do recognize that if my recipes are delicious enough they could cause overconsumption.

Food Augmenters

Getting a creamy texture in a ketogenic recipe is a breeze, but chewy, crispy and crunchy present much more of a challenge. To get these we will need judicious use of augmenters. Getting acquainted with the following list of low carbohydrate augmenting ingredients will help you explore and create new recipes.

- Emulsifiers
  - Soy lecithin
  - Eggs
- Chewy
  - Chicory inulin
  - Beef gelatin
  - Cured meats
  - Guar Gum
- Crispy
  - Freeze dried berries
  - Roasted leaves (kale, chard, seaweed)
- Crunchy
  - Bacon
  - Pork rinds
  - Insects
  - Nuts (use sparingly)
  - Cocoa nibs

IV. MY KETO EXPERIENCE ON THE TRAIL

14. Keto on the Appalachian Trail

Planning and Packing for the AT

The air was earthy and fresh. Our evening was illuminated by the exotic guest of light from the other side of the earth. Having bounced off the moon, it dropped to the fluffy bed of clouds below us and bounded up again, catching the fresh dew on the grass and tickling the pale lichen on the oaks. We were in a gallery of magician's mirrors and an amphitheater of the heavens. Sitting atop Mt Tamalpais, the golden tresses of the hills known as the "seven sisters" undulated in the cool ocean breeze below us. We were alive. We were in love with one another and the outdoors. The world was our playground. I asked her to be marry me.

Four years, and many adventures later, we were two tiny specks picking our way through the glacier-carved, boulder-strewn expanse of California's Desolation Wilderness. The question of backpacking food was forefront in my mind. Jess was four months pregnant with our first child. Long before this child was conceived, we had planned our first family adventure. The destination and scope of the adventure would be determined by the season in which our child would be born and the vigor of mother and child.

Our daughter Zia was due in late January, she would be 10 weeks old in mid-April, too late for a New Zealand trek, too early for any mountains in the west, but just right for starting the Appalachian trail.

By any modern standard, the fact that Jess would be contemplating a long-distance hike at 10 weeks post-partum was heroic. Uncertain of how her body would handle the rigors of the trail, we wanted to keep her pack as light as possible. This meant I would be carrying most of the load.

Bringing a baby meant carrying a little more weight. Zia herself would weigh 13lbs when we started and 16lbs by the time we finished our hike two months later. We had chosen a larger heavier shelter and exchanged our shared down quilt for separate sleeping bags, so I wouldn't be woken every time Zia needed to nurse. With these changes and a few diapers (less thanks to Elimination Communication techniques) and warm clothes for the family our total family base weight was 49lbs including Zia[175,176]. Add another four pounds to keep two liters of water on hand to ensure Jess stayed sufficiently hydrated to produce a steady supply of milk for our growing adventurer and the total family pack weight was now 53lbs.

Split among the two of us, an individual weight of ~27lbs wasn't bad, but we wouldn't be dividing the weight evenly. Not having had the opportunity to carry our growing child for 10 months of pregnancy, I supposed this was my chance to pitch in. If Jess carried Zia and the water, my pack would be 46lbs… plus all the food.

Food would be the biggest part of our pack weight.

As we passed through the fragrant shade of a fir grove, Jess offered the classic biological strategy to an upcoming period of caloric deficit: "You could just get fat ahead of time and live off your fat stores" she said. Despite Jess' breastfeeding we were both aware that mine would still be the biggest stomach to fill on the trail. At 190lbs and 8% body fat my caloric consumption while reclining on a lounge chair all day had been measured as 2114kcal at the DEXAfit lab in San Francisco. This value is known is the resting metabolic rate or RMR. The metabolic equivalent value for backpacking (metabolic equivalent, or MET, of 7) predicted an expenditure of 635kcal/hr. Multiply this by eight hours of backpacking and this added 5,080kcal to my daily caloric need for a total of 7,194kcal.

I knew from my recent DEXA scans at DEXAfit San Francisco, that I had 18lbs of fat on my body, 13lbs was essential which left me with 5lbs of fat to spare. For each pound of human fat, approximately 25% would be water and protein and 75% would be actual fat[3][177][178]. At 9kcal/g this would give me 3000 kcal per pound of fat and a total of 15,000kcal. This was enough calories to supply two full days of hiking 8hrs a day.

Once this fat was gone, my body would only be left with my hard-earned muscle to burn. I could forestall this by fattening up ahead of time, a strategy my vanity made decidedly unattractive, not to mention the problem of hunger. But even with the extra fat stores, I was still at risk of losing muscle mass as some studies on caloric restriction in overweight individuals have shown.

As we squeezed under a huge sequoia lying across the trail, her pregnant belly now noticeably protruding, our thoughts turned to feeding Jess on our first family adventure.

---

[3] A pound of pure fat would be 3,500kcal but fat on an actual human is stored as adipose tissue which is composed of 15% cellular water and protein and thus would only hold 2,975kcal. While this number is well established, there is debate as to whether a reduction of caloric intake of 3,500 will actually result in 1lb of fat loss because human rates of fat burning varies.

Later Jessica's post-partum breastfeeding RMR would be measured in the same DEXAfit San Francisco lab as mine at 1418kcal/day. The same 7 MET value predicted an additional 4,784kcal expenditure for eight hours a day of backpacking. This put her total daily caloric need at 6,202kcal and the total daily family caloric need at 13,396kcal. Although we were confident that our resting metabolic rates were accurate, we knew the expenditure during hiking would range greatly according to the terrain and pack weight, but one things seemed clear, we would need a lot of food.

On a typical diet of 30%fat, 15% protein and 65% carbohydrates, this 13,396kcal would consist of 447 grams of fat, 502 grams of protein and 2,177 grams of carbohydrate for a total weight of 6.9lbs per day. In reality, this food would be heavier thanks to packaging, water and fiber.

Just three days of the family's food would bring my pack weight up to 74 pounds. Five days of food would bring the pack weight up to an absurd 88lbs.

I knew the solution to fueling our family adventure was fat. I had experimented with the effect of the ketogenic diet on my cycling performance a year before and had excellent results. I had been looking for good ketogenic backpacking recipes but had found none. I would have to come up with them myself.

In the year leading up to our Appalachian trail hike, I experimented with ketogenic foods in the kitchen and on the trail. Each backpacking trip we went on was a test, there were a few delicious successes and many failed attempts to make mayonnaise on the trail without fresh eggs. As our child grew in the womb, so did my menu of ketogenic backpacking recipes.

I hope these recipes provide you with as much energy and enjoyment as they have provided me and my family.

Getting into Ketosis: Month One

I started the ketogenic diet three and a half months before hitting the trail to give me plenty of time to enter ketosis and test recipes along the way. I began recording my daily food intake using the MyFitnessPal app on February 5th, 2017, one week after my daughter was born.

At the same time, I began measuring my fasting morning levels of both types of ketone bodies. I used a blood drop from a finger prick to measure my blood beta-hydroxybutyrate levels using the Precision One-Touch Ultra and I exhaled into the Ketonix breath acetone monitor to measure my acetoacetate levels.

Once a month I visited the DEXAfit lab in San Francisco for a suite of measurements. This included 1) the gold standard of body composition, dual x-ray absorptiometry (DEXA) which calculated the precise amount of bone, fat and a lean mass in my body; 2) infrared volume measurement of the circumferences of my arms, legs, torso and neck; 3) my resting metabolic rate; 4) and my respiratory exchange ratio (RER). This latter measurement revealed the extent to which I was burning fat vs carbohydrates at rest.

For three days I stayed on my normal mixed diet to establish a baseline. During these three days my average intake was 4093kcal, 51% fat, 35% carbs and 15% protein. This was a high fat diet averaging 229g of fat per day but not a low carb diet as it contained 362g of carbs. It was also a high protein and high fiber diet with an average of145g of protein and 102g of fiber per day. I had spent the prior four months on a diet restricted to ~2,700kcal/day with a similar nutrient ratio.

My average morning blood ketone levels after each of these three days was 0.2mmol/L and my breath acetone average was 71. Both values showed no significant ketone production.

On February 8th, 2017 I visited the DEXAfit lab. I weighed 191.2lbs, with 17.9lbs of fat, 161.1lbs of muscle and 8.0lbs of bone for a percent body fat of 9.6%. My resting metabolic rate was 1686kcal, this was substantially lower than measurements three months prior and was the result of having reduced my caloric intake to decrease my body fat for the last three months. My metabolism was burning 56% fat and 44% carbs at rest with a respiratory exchange ratio of 0.83.

After leaving the lab I began the ketogenic diet as follows: I restricted my carbohydrate intake to <20 grams per day, kept my protein intake <1g/lb of lean mass and ate as much fat as needed to feel full. On most days I had a ketogenic broth or other hot beverage on my morning hike carrying Zia, cheese and salami for lunch and tested out new recipes for dinner.

One month later, my blood ketone levels (BHOB) had crossed the 1mmol mark of nutritional ketosis only once. My average blood beta-hydroxybutyrate level for the month was 0.5mmol and my breath acetone level was 71. I felt fine, with none of the side effects of keto-adaptation others had mentioned such as fatigue, mental fogginess or light headedness but I wasn't producing ketones.

My average intake for the month was 4,807kcal, 392g of fat, 17g of carbohydrate and 123grams of protein per day. I had eaten more than 20g of carbohydrate on only three occasions and on these days I had eaten 34, 21 and 28g. My protein intake had exceeded 161 only once at 167g on February 23rd, 2017. I had followed a ketogenic diet carefully, but I wasn't producing ketones. What was wrong?

My body composition results were unrevealing, as I was nearly the same as before at 186lbs and 10% fat with 18.5lbs of fat, 158lbs of lean mass and 8.0lbs of bone. This 3.1lb drop in lean mass could easily be accounted for by the depletion of my glycogen stores on the ketogenic diet. The 0.6lb increase in my fat was all in my torso but very little of it in and around the organs. All in all, these changes were very small and could not reliable be distinguished from measurement variation.

My DEXAfit metabolic results after this first month, gave the clue as to what might have been happening. My resting metabolic rate had jumped up by 367kal to 2053kal and my % fat burning had decreased substantially down to 33% fat and 77% carbs with a respiratory exchange ratio of 0.93! How was I burning more carbs now that I was eating practically no carbohydrates (17g/day)? There was only one answer: gluconeogenesis.

My brain and body were relying on blood sugar produced in the liver by a process known as gluconeogenesis. I can't be entirely sure where this glucose was coming from, but I suspect it was mostly from my dietary protein intake. Studies on fasting show that up to 20% of new glucose is made from the glycerol backbone of fats (triglycerides) during fasting and much of the remaining glucose is recycled from lactate via the fat-powered Cori cycle but it is still unclear what proportion of various substrates are used to provide glucose on a ketogenic diet[42,179-182]. My protein intake might have been high enough to keep liver glycogen and oxaloacetate levels sufficient to prevent the production of ketones and reduce my body's fat burning. This drop in fat burning was a surprising result as the 1gram of protein/lb of lean mass calculation has resulted in nutritional ketosis for others[2].

Getting into Ketosis: Month Two

In the following week I had two morning blood ketone reading of 1.1mmol but the rest were all 0.7mmol or less and my average for the week was 0.8mmol/L. At the same time, I was started taking blood ketone readings of Jess who was breastfeed but not eating a strict ketogenic diet and hers where through the roof at 1.3, 2.4 and 5mmol! She was eating the ketogenic backpacking recipes I was testing out in the evening as well as the hot beverages in the morning, but she was not restricting carbohydrates and was eating foods like chocolate, almond butter and rye seed toast.

Meanwhile my average daily intake for the last week had been 3606kcal, 351g of fat, 15g of carbohydrates and 96g of protein.

I was jealous. Was breastfeeding giving Jess a superpower to produce ketones? Why did my body prefer to make sugar from protein instead of producing ketones? After thinking it over for a week I decided to cut my protein intake from 161g (1g/lb of lean mass) to 72g starting March 15th, 2017. This amount was 10% above the 65g minimum protein intake for my body size recommended by the World Health Organization using their calculation of 0.36g/lb of total body mass. I had been hesitant to do this before because I was concerned that decreasing my protein intake would result in the loss of lean mass. This change took some recalibration of my diet and was especially tricky when trying to estimate the protein content of uncommon foods such as slow cooked Mangalitsa pork skin with adipose.

I started off with a day of only 33 grams of protein, mostly by accident because I didn't tally my food until the end of the day, and I was afraid to eat too much protein. I was rewarded the next day with a fasted morning blood beta-hydroxybutyrate level of 1.4mmol/L. From that point on my levels were consistently above 1mmol and the average for the next two weeks was 1.2mmol/L with my highest reading at 5.7mmol/L!

After a week of consistently high readings I was confident I was in nutritional ketosis. In addition to my morning measurements I began measuring my blood ketone levels after specific meals to test the ketogenic effect of the recipes. I found I was able to slightly increase either my daily protein or carbohydrate intake so long as any given maintained a Wilder ratio over 3:1. My carbohydrate and protein intakes never exceeded 54 and 124grams respectively, and never this high in both on the same day.

Previously I had made the mistake of concentrating all my protein to one or two meals and apparently this had been enough to stimulate gluconeogenesis.

On April 5th, 2017, now at the end of the second month of the ketogenic diet and having finally produced ketones, I returned to DEXAfit San Francisco, excited to see the results.

My body composition results were potentially skewed by a side effect of the ketogenic diet: slowed intestinal transit time. As long as I can remember I have had a very rapid intestinal transit time and thus have been prone to diarrhea. In remember investigating this in college by eating sesame seeds with a meal as a tracer, then seeing them in my stool six hours later. The ketogenic diet had slowed me down to a normal pace and I went from several stools a day to once a day or even once every other day. Before each DEXA scan I fasted for 15hours overnight and had my scan at the same time the following morning. Usually I would have at least one bowel movement but this time I didn't.

My weight and body composition were nearly the same at 186.9lbs and 9.9% fat. This consisted of 21lbs of fat, 161lbs of lean mass and 7.9lbs of bone. I had gained 2.5lbs of fat with 2lbs of it in my torso but I had also gained 3.2lbs of lean mass in my torso. The lean portion of this was likely due to stool content as previous testing comparing fasted and fed states had revealed similar changes in torso lean mass.

My metabolic results were finally showing nutritional ketosis with a respiratory exchange ratio of 0.75 indicated 84% fat burning at rest! My resting metabolic rate had bumped up to 2114kcal/day, now 428kcal and 25% higher than my pre-ketogenic level of 1686kcal/day two months prior. This may have been due to my increase in caloric intake in this second month, up to 4,602kcal from 4087kcal in the first month, 4093kcal in the three days before my baseline measurement and ~2,700 in the four months prior to that. My activity level had not changed dramatically in this time period although I was hiking a few miles every morning with newborn baby Zia starting January 29th, 2017 Overall, I was working out less than I had in the four months I spent eating ~2,700kcal. By the end of two months I was eating 509kcal more than when I started, and my metabolism had elevated by 428kcal.

As my stores of blood ketone test strips began to run low, I started measuring my blood glucose and seeing the correlation between it and my blood ketones. I found that if my blood glucose was below 90mg/dL, my blood beta-hydroxybutyrate was over 1mmol/L.

Hitting the Trail in Ketosis

My entire time on the ketogenic diet I remained free of commonly reported negative side effects. I had been diligent to maintain our fluid and electrolyte levels and we divided our food into 4-5 meals throughout the day. My sodium intake had consistently been >3,000mg per day and closer to 8,000mg on sweaty days when I was drinking 10+ liters of water.

I measured my fasted morning glucose every few days and my blood ketones once a week. My ketone levels ranged from 0.6 to 5.1mmol with an average of 1.8mmol/L and my glucose levels ranged from 77mg/dL to 105mg/dL with an average of 91mg/dL.

After a few days of packing and preparing resupply boxes we started our Appalachian Trail section hike northbound at Rockfish Gap on April 16th, 2017. I continued to experience consistent energy levels and had no negative side effects.

Shortly after starting our hike, news of the "family hiking with a baby" and the "dad who eats only fat" quickly spread and people greeted us on the trail as if we were old friends. My willingness to talk about my diet quickly validated my trail name "Keto." The trail name Sherpa was suggested but it had already been given to Derrick Quirin who was hiking the entire trail that year with his wife Bekah "Kanga" and one-year-old baby Ellie "Roo." We tried to give our own daughter Zia the trail name "Leech" on account of her sucking the milk and energy out of Jess but this name was repeatedly rejected, and Jess started going by "Leche" and Zia by "Chupaleche", translated "The Milk Sucker."

We both enjoyed the food we had packed but quickly found that the 10,000kcal/day I had packed for the family was far more than we needed. This was still less than the 13,396kcal estimate from the metabolic equivalent value for backpacking. Perhaps this was because the section we were hiking was less steep or our pace was slower because of stopping to nurse Zia.

We looked forward to the meals but rarely found ourselves hungry. I soon began sending things back or throwing them out. We consistently showed up at a resupply with a day or two of extra food. Much effort in food packing and a lot of good olive oil was wasted.

In the end, our pace on the trail was not limited by energy but by the aches and pains of adapting to hiking all day. We had planned to start out at 8 miles per day, but after a few days we were feeling antsy after arriving at camp at 3pm and picked it up to 13 miles per day.

Soon Jess' knees were hurting and soon after our feet hit the cruel rocks of Pennsylvania. Feet and knees were ongoing issues, and Jess was hit hardest having had little time after giving birth to prepare her body. Frequent stopping to nurse our growing daughter also checked our pace and I did my best to quell my restless spirit and settle in and enjoy the ride. The various orthopedic challenges we experienced tested my on-trail physical therapy skills and we reached Dalton, MA sixty days and 707 miles later on June 14th, 2017. We had average 13 miles per day, 12 per day when including our six zero days with a median mileage of 14.

Once a week I did two sets each of the same four upper body strength exercises: 1) handstand pushups, 2) pullups; 3) pushups; and 4) body weight rows.
I did not do any specific lower body strength training.

I continued the ketogenic diet uninterrupted all the way through our Appalachian trail section hike and after, ending 143 days, nearly 5 months later on July 2nd, 2017.

On the way to a wedding in Minnesota I was scheduled to stopped by DEXAfit Minneapolis for my final measurements. We had missed an early morning connection flight thanks to me taking a nap by a self-playing piano in the Chicago O-Hare airport and as a result I walked into the lab the next afternoon having fasted for 23 hours vs the usual 15 hours.

My DEXA results showed I was nearly the same weight at 186.5lbs but my body composition had shifted in an unfavorable direction. There was no change in my arms, but my legs lost 1.2lbs of muscle and gained 1.3lbs of fat. Apparently that heavy pack hadn't built any muscle after all. Despite this increase in fat in my legs, they looked leaner. This may have been due to an increase in intramuscular fat and decrease in superficial fat known to occur with long duration endurance training.

The largest and least trustworthy changes were seen in my torso which lost 4lbs of lean mass and gained 1.9lbs of fat compared to my last measurement. This torso lean change be attributed to the fact that my last measurement contained bowel contents and this measurement did not. But the fat mass increase was likely a true body fat increase.

When compared to my original, pre-ketogenic diet I had gained 6.4lbs of fat and lost 5.6lbs of lean mass with most of these changes occurring during my time on the Appalachian trail.

My respiratory exchange ratio was off the charts at 0.72, showed I was burning 95% fat at rest. However, my metabolism had slowed down by 11% to 1892kcal/day. This is similar to the basal metabolic rate drop of 10% that has been found in the research to accompany long duration aerobic exercise.

Summary

Despite diligent carbohydrate restriction I did not produce substantial ketones until I reduced my protein intake. During my entire time on the ketogenic diet I did not experience any negative side effects. My energy levels felt constant and I never had hiker hunger. I lost lean mass, and this can be attributed to a combination of glycogen loss seen in the first month of entering ketosis and true lean mass loss resulting from long distance hiking without sufficient strength training. I overpacked in food and ended up gaining fat along the trail. After rising initially, my metabolism dropped back down after the hike.

Without having done a similar hike on a different diet I had nothing to compare the results to, but generally I was happy with the performance of the ketogenic diet. Still, I felt the pace we had set as a family was not testing the limits of my metabolic system and I was itching to get out on my own and push myself to the limit.

Appalachian Trail Figures

Notes:

- I began eating the ketogenic diet immediately after the 2/8/17 measurement.
- I reduced my protein intake and started producing significant blood ketones after the 3/8/17 measurement.

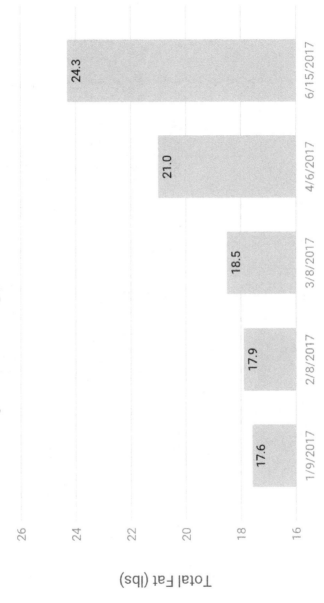

6.4lb Increase in Body Fat on Ketogenic Diet

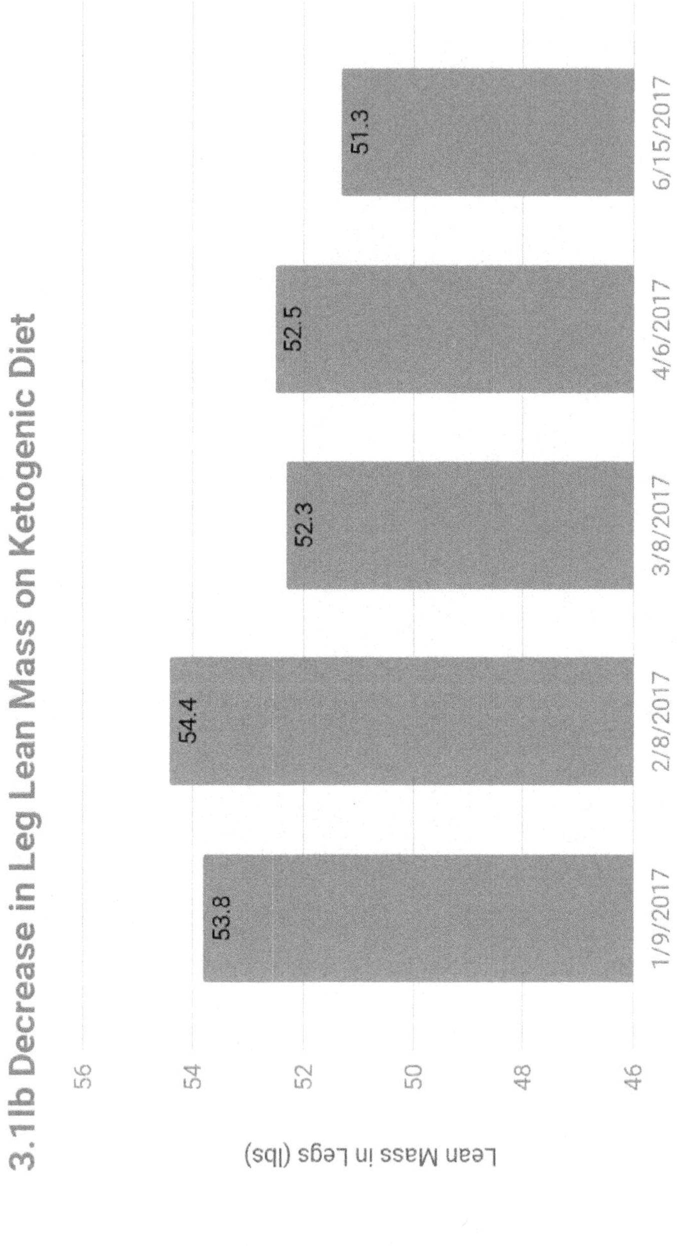
3.1lb Decrease in Leg Lean Mass on Ketogenic Diet
Lean Mass in Legs (lbs)
56
54
52
50
48
46
53.8
54.4
52.3
52.5
51.3
1/9/2017
2/8/2017
3/8/2017
4/6/2017
6/15/2017

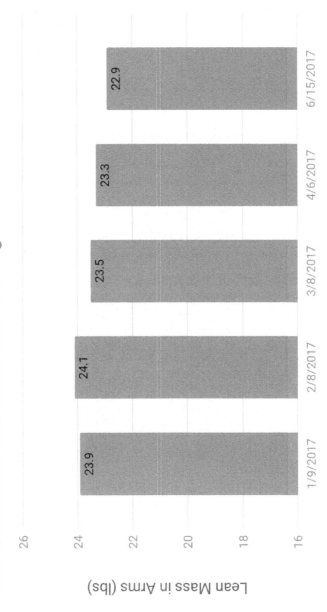

1.2lb Decrease in Arm Lean Mass on Ketogenic Diet

Lean Mass in Arms (lbs)

Date	Value
1/9/2017	23.9
2/8/2017	24.1
3/8/2017	23.5
4/6/2017	23.3
6/15/2017	22.9

Notes:

- Throughout the measurement period I completed the same upper body strength training session only once per week.

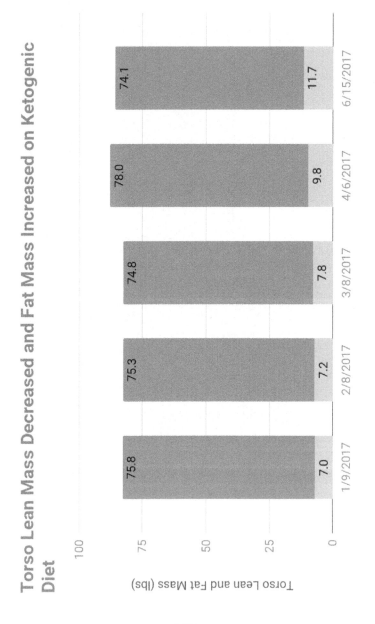

Torso Lean Mass Decreased and Fat Mass Increased on Ketogenic Diet

Notes:
- I fasted 15hrs before the first four measurements. I passed a stool during this fast on the first the measurements but not before 4/6/17. The increased torso lean mas can be attributed to the presence of stool.
- I fasted for 23hrs before the 6/15/17 measurement.

0.7cm Increase in Waist Circumference on Ketogenic Diet

Bar chart showing Waist Circumference at Narrowest Point (cm) across dates:
- 1/8/17 12:30: 82.9
- 2/8/17 12:30: 83.9
- 3/8/17 12:00: 85.6
- 4/10/17 12:00: 85.0
- 6/13/17 16:00: 84.6

Y-axis: Waist Circumference at Narrowest Point (cm), ranging from 82 to 86.

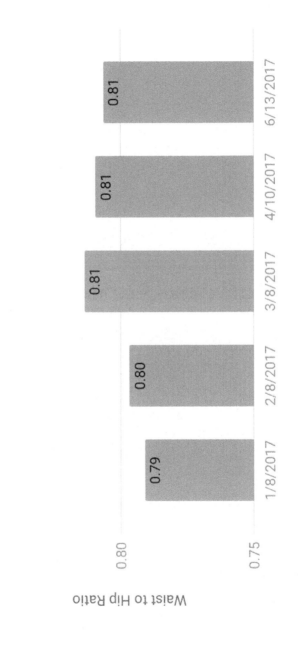

0.02 Increase in Waist to Hip Ratio on Ketogenic Diet

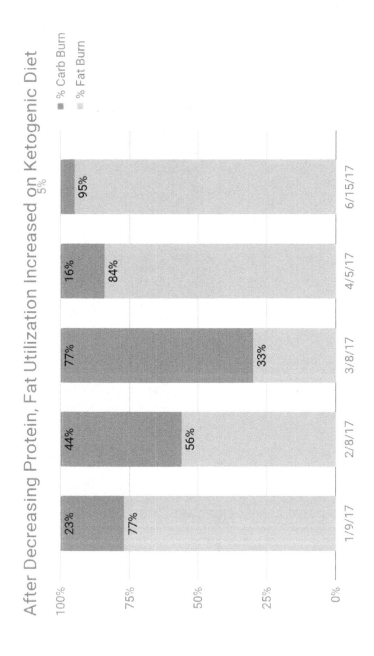

After Decreasing Protein, Fat Utilization Increased on Ketogenic Diet

No Clear Trends in Body Circumference on Ketogenic Diet

Circumference (cm)

Date	1/8/2017	2/8/2017	3/8/2017	4/10/2017	6/13/2017
	125.9	124.5	122.7	122.5	123.1
	109.9	108.8	109.4	110.5	108.4
	104.8	105.3	105.2	105.0	104.9
	80.0	80.4	78.3	78.8	80.5
	71.2	70.4	71.8	72.2	73.4

Notes:
- Red: Sum of both thigh circumferences
- Purple: Chest circumference

107

- Blue: Hip Circumference at Widest Part
- Yellow: Sum of calf circumferences at widest point at axillary fold
- Green: Sum of arm circumferences
- I hike the Appalachian Trail from April 16th,2017 to June 14th, 2017.

Fasted Morning Blood Ketone Levels Over Time

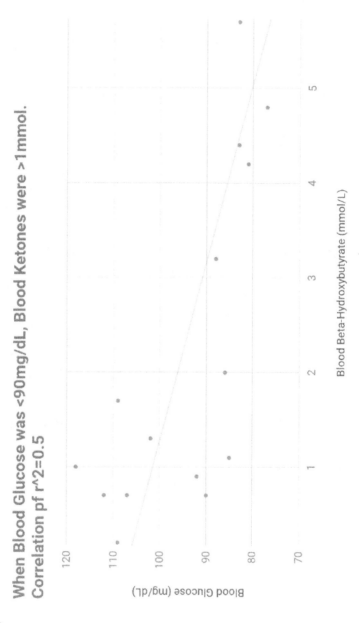

When Blood Glucose was <90mg/dL, Blood Ketones were >1mmol. Correlation pf r^2=0.5

Blood Glucose (mg/dL)

Blood Beta-Hydroxybutyrate (mmol/L)

Notes:
- These measurements were taken from 3/21/17 to 7/2/17 and many were taken on the Appalachian Trail.

- These blood glucose and ketone measurements were taken simultaneously.
- These measurements were taken at various points throughout the day, some in fasted and others in fed states.

Most High Blood Ketone Measurements Occurred When Prior Day's Protein Was <92g

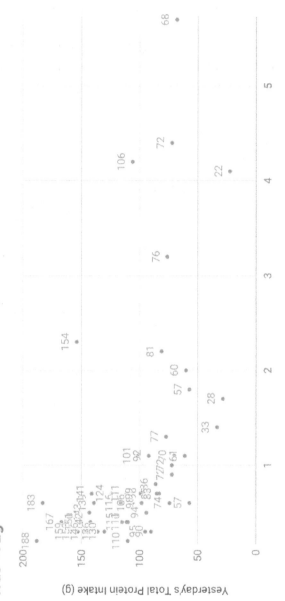

Fasted Morning Beta-Hydroxybutyrate (mmol/L)

Yesterday's Total Protein Intake (g)

Most High Blood Ketone Measurements Occurred When My Prior Day's Protein Intake in Grams Was <50% of My Total Body Lean Mass in Pounds

Notes:

- These measurements were taken between 2/8/17 and 4/6/17, before starting the Appalachian Trail on 4/16/17.

Fasted Morning Blood Ketones Correlated Positively (r^2= 0.4) With Previous Day's Wilder Ratio

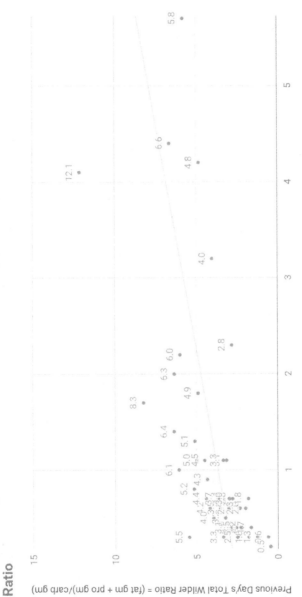

Previous Day's Total Wilder Ratio = (fat gm)/(pro gm + carb gm)

Fasted Morning Beta-Hydroxybutyrate (mmol/L)

No Correlation Between Fasted Morning Blood Ketones and Previous Day Carbohydrate Intake

Notes:

- These measurements were taken between 2/8/17 and 4/6/17, before starting the Appalachian Trail on 4/16/17.

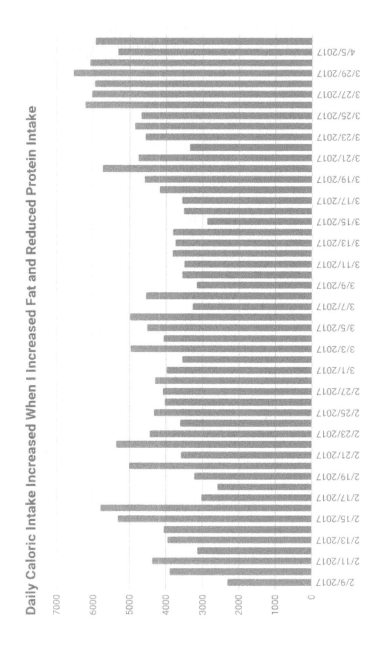

Daily Caloric Intake Increased When I Increased Fat and Reduced Protein Intake

118

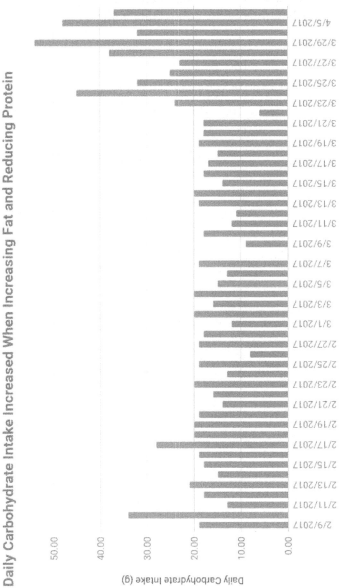

Daily Carbohydrate Intake Increased When Increasing Fat and Reducing Protein

Notes:

- These measurements were taken between 2/8/17 and 4/6/17, before starting the Appalachian Trail on 4/16/17.

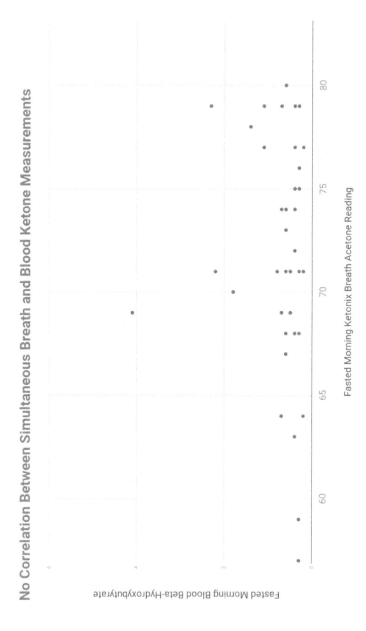

Notes:

- These measurements were taken between 2/8/17 and 4/6/17, before starting the Appalachian Trail on 4/16/17.

15. Keto in the Whites

The first part of this story consists of the details of planning for my ultralight speed-packing trip in the White Mountains of New Hampshire. Scroll to the end to find out what happened.

Going fast, but not too fast.
Carbohydrate depletion impairs sprint speed and may impair peak aerobic capacity[183,184]. You need carbs to perform your best in repeated bouts of explosive movement, i.e. weightlifting, combat and field sports. But you don't need carbs to do slower things like hike or bike at a moderate pace[185]. A ketogenic diet is the perfect way to maximize fat burning and lower pack weight on a bike tour or backpacking trip over moderate terrain. I hiked 707miles of the Appalachian Trail on a ketogenic diet carrying a pack full of food and gear for myself, my wife and my 11-week-old daughter, and sometimes carrying her too. But what about hiking fast up mountains? Is speed-packing too fast for keto? Do you need carbs to bag peaks?

I decided to test the limits of the ketogenic diet on an aggressive speed-packing trip in the White Mountains of New Hampshire.

Crunching the numbers
A study on elite cyclists found that a month of eating only 10% of calories from carbohydrates increased the amount of work that could be done from fat alone from their former range of 90-540kcal/hr up to 660-1000kcal/hr[11]. Weighing 180lb and carrying a 16lb pack, I would need to burn around 600 kcal/hr which was well within the range of the

keto-adapted cyclists but above the range of the carb-eating cyclists. I recently tested my respiratory exchange ratio at DEXAFIT Minneapolis and found I was burning 95% fat at rest. Would I be able to burn fat at a high enough rate to fuel me up the steep climbs of the White Mountains of New Hampshire?

How much should I eat?
My calculations predicted a whopping daily expenditure of 7906kcal; 6014kcal from hiking for 10 hours plus my resting metabolic rate of 1892 from my recent test at DEXAFIT Minneapolis. I decided to bring only 5,000kcal/day and burn body fat to fuel the rest for three reasons:
– Prolonged endurance exercise blunts my appetite
– Prolonged endurance exercise impairs my digestion
– My experience hiking the Appalachian Trail makes me suspicious that the caloric expenditure estimates above are too high.

I knew from my latest DEXA scan from DEXAFIT Minneapolis that I was carrying 14lbs of unessential fat. The ketogenic diet would allow me to tap into this 42,000kcal of fat and burn it at a rapid rate. If I did burn 8,000kcal/day for 4 days and eat 5,000kca/day I would lose pound of fat a day. Why carry it in your pack when you already have it on your body?

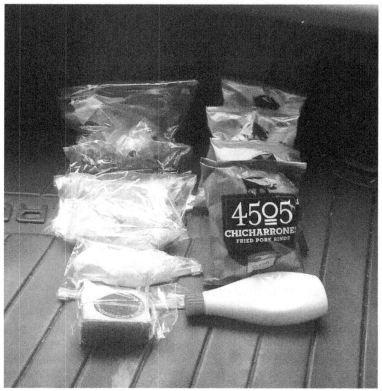

My meal plan
I decided to go stove-less to reduce weight and save time.
In the heat of midsummer, hot food wasn't missed.

I planned to hike for four days and eat five meals a day,
about 1,000kcal each. Breaking it up this way ensured I
would have enough bile to absorb each meal.

I packed a total of 20,490kcal, weighing 6lbs with a
combined Wilder ratio of 4.4 and a total cost of $83.85. I
could have cut costs with cheaper ingredients, but I opted
for high quality fuel.

Here is the menu I packed:

Food	Kcal	Wilder	Fat (g)	Carb (g)	Pro (g)	kcal/oz	$
Thai Cashew Cream	5445	5.3	548	72	32	217	$11.29
Pomegranite Jetpack	1696	4.0	171	42	1	211	$7.37
Absolute Black Fudge	2858	3.6	305	52	32	200	$12.97
Lardican	4148	4.3	418	0	98	211	$17.09
Manchego and Cheese	2800	3.9	276	0	70	156	$9.73
Chicharrones and Mayo	3543	5.0	363	0	72	194	$25.39

My Gear

Instead of bringing a lot of ultralight gear, I followed the strategy of only bringing things I would absolutely need. I used the Clark hammock and rainfly I already had instead of buying a lighter shelter. I brought two battery packs to ensure I would be able to capture all my data on Strava. A pair of shorts for hiking, thermals for sleeping and no rain gear. If I am hiking fast I stay warm, if I bring the rain gear I just sweat in it.

I anticipated that orthopedic problems would be my limiting factor, so I planned to rely heavily on my trekking poles, tape key areas and take a high dose of fish oil.

Here is my pack weighing 16lbs including food:

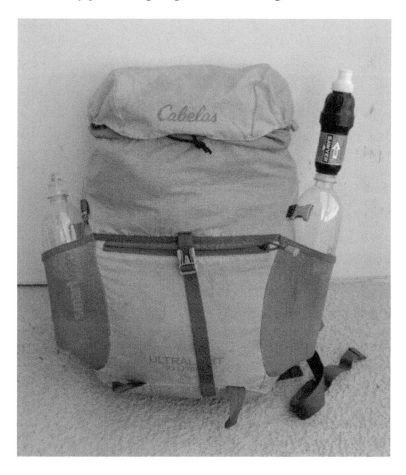

Here are the contents of my pack excluding food:

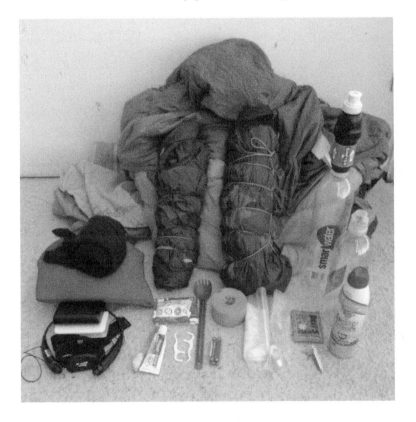

Here is the spreadsheet of my pack contents showing the weight of each item:

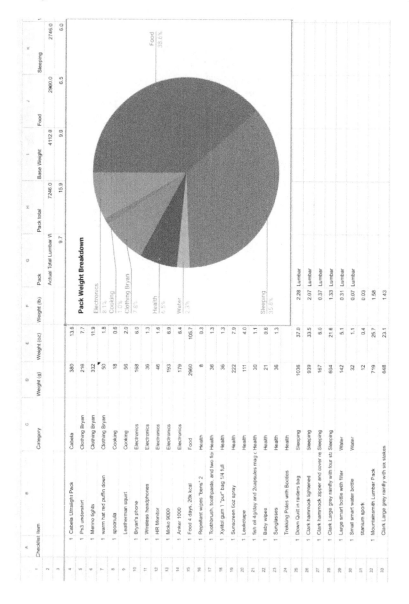

	Checklist Item	Category	Weight (g)	Weight (oz)	Weight (lb)	Pack
			Actual Total Lumbar W	Pack total	Base Weight	Food	Sleeping
			9.7	15.9	9.0	6.5	6.0
			7246.0	4112.0	2960.0	2746.0	
1	Cabela Ultralight Pack	Cabela	380	13.6		
1	Pk3 undershirt	Clothing Bryan	216	7.7		
1	Merino tights	Clothing Bryan	332	11.9		
1	warm hat red puffin down	Clothing Bryan	50	1.8		
1	spoonula	Cooking	18	0.6		
1	Leatherman squirt	Cooking	56	2.0		
1	Bryan's phone	Electronics	168	6.0		
1	Wireless headphones	Electronics	36	1.3		
1	HR Monitor	Electronics	46	1.6		
1	Moko 9000	Electronics	193	6.9		
1	Anker 1000	Electronics	179	6.4		
1	Food 4 days, 20k kcal	Food	2960	105.7		
1	Repellant wipes "bens" 2	Health	8	0.3		
1	Toothbrush, toothpaste, and two flos	Health	36	1.3		
1	Xylitol gum 1 "pour" bag 1/4 full	Health	36	1.3		
1	Sunscreen 6oz spray	Health	222	7.9		
1	Leukotape	Health	111	4.0		
1	fish oil 4g/day and 2capsules mag c	Health	30	1.1		
1	Baby wipes	Health	21	0.8		
1	Sunglasses	Health	36	1.3		
1	Trekking Poles with Booties	Health	1036	37.0		
1	Down Quilt in raiders bag	Sleeping	939	33.5	2.28 Lumbar	
1	Clark hammock lightened	Sleeping	167	6.0	2.07 Lumbar	
1	Clark hammock zipper and cover re	Sleeping	604	21.6	0.37 Lumbar	
1	Clark Large grey rainfly with four sti	Sleeping	142	5.1	1.33 Lumbar	
1	Large smart bottle with filter	Water	32	1.1	0.31 Lumbar	
1	Small smart water bottle	Water	12	0.4	0.07 Lumbar	
1	titanium spork		719	25.7	0.03	
1	Mountainsmith Lumbar Pack		648	23.1	1.58	
1	Clark Large grey rainfly with six stakes				1.43	

Pack Weight Breakdown

Food 38.6%
Electronics 8.1%
Cooking 1.0%
Clothing Bryan 7.8%
Health 6.5%
Water 2.3%
Sleeping 35.8%

The Results

Keto worked. I had tons of energy. I attacked slippery steep climbs, charged through ankle-deep mud in alpine bogs and raced from peak to peak for 12 hours straight. Strava recorded 51 miles, 16,913ft of elevation and 10,881kcal burned in two days. I ate about 3,000kcal each day and never got hungry leaving a deficit of about 8,665kcal, or 2.8lbs of fat burned in 2 days. My body burned its fat stores in a bonfire that fueled an epic adventure.

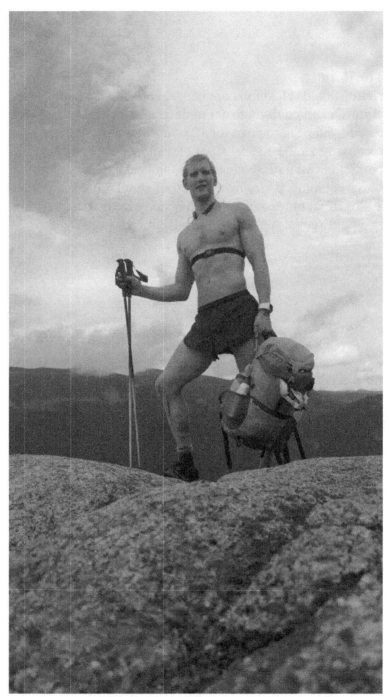

White Mountains Day One: June 30th, 2017

Breath in, two, three, four, breath out six, seven, eight, nine ten. Orange barrels blurred by, walls of dark foliage leaned in and the first drops began to burst on the windshield. By the time I parked at the Basin Trailhead and put away my Muse meditation headband, the roof was drumming with a steady rain. I hadn't planned for this.

A dull tingling informed me that my right leg planned on waking up a little later than the rest of me. I pulled the reluctant leg back across the center console and strapped on my HR monitor to measure my heart rate variability (HRV). Three minutes later I was advised to take a rest day.

Despite 90 minutes of calm breathing on yesterday's drive, my HRV was 70 and my HF was 506, numbers well below my norms in the mid-80s and 2,000s indicating my nervous system was stressed. This was the first day of my four-day solo assault on the White Mountains. At least my metabolic system was in the right place, last night's blood ketone levels were very high at 5.0mmol/L.

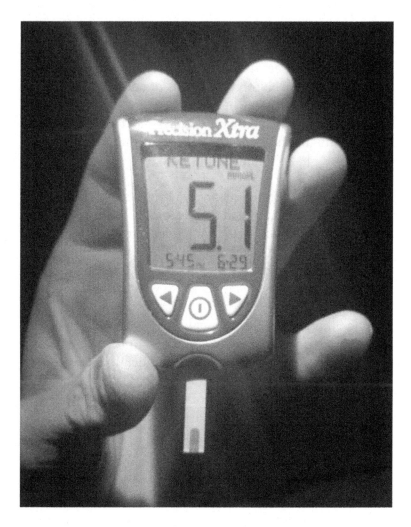

Two weeks prior I finished a 707-mile section hike on the Appalachian trail with my wife and 11-week-old daughter. I had carried a 50-80lbs pack, depending on the amount of food and whether I was carrying the baby. Without the ketogenic diet my pack would have been heavier, or we would have had to resupply every few days, or worse lose some of the lean mass I had worked for years to accumulate. My feet had hurt but my energy had never flagged on the ketogenic diet and I wondered what I would be capable of with a lighter pack.

Now with a pack weighing 16lbs I felt like I was floating down the trail. I relished the feeling of walking without pain, washed in green, drawn into the mountains by a heady redolence of pine and moist earth. Then my wrist started to hurt. I taped it with a technique I learned at a Mulligan course years before. The pain went away. So far so good.

Like a playground bully, the trail dared me to climb up the slide… then poured water down it. I gained 2,500 feet of wet rock and mud in 2.5 miles, then sailed along the high ridge another 1,200 feet to Mt Lafayette, gaining the admiration of more than one summer camp hiking group and a growing ache around the kneecaps.

I ducked out of the wind and began taping my knees, better to stay ahead of this pain. I wasn't hungry or thirsty, but I thought it prudent to stay ahead of those things too. I crunched clouds of pork skin with stiff peaks of mayo and then floated down sheets of wet granite. More than once my feet flew down ahead of me. Each time I picked myself back up, grateful for no severe injury. The day rolled on, the trail passed under my feet, the trees returned, as did the rain. My knees were feeling better, but there was a new sensation in my Achilles.

Ambient temps were in the 50s and the water felt colder, but I waded into the Saco river for a pre-slumber ablution on the premise that after 27 miles and 8,736ft of elevation some cryotherapy was in order. After a seven-minute feast of shredded beef in lard followed by chunks of peanut cocoa fudge and two magnesium tablets, I rocked off to sleep in my Clark Jungle Hammock as falling drops typed on my rainfly.

White Mountains Day Two: July 1st, 2017

And so my day of presidents began. On the stairs to Webster, Jackson, and Pierce, a wall of roots and wet rocks greeted me that blurred the definitions of hiking and rock climbing. After a few scoops of MCT rich blend I call Pomegranate Jetpack, I skated the slimy puncheons of an Alpine Bog, then discussed the weather with the hostess at Mizpah Spring Hut while savoring water I hadn't had to filter.

On Eisenhower the weather turned.

At first it was a touch of rain, and a dimming of the lights. But steady curtains of moisture began to fall, and it was real rain by the time I reached the Lake of the Clouds Hut. More pork clouds and mayo and a sobering check of the forecast. Severe thunderstorm warning for the rest of the afternoon. Mt Washington was 1.5miles away, then 7 miles of exposed trail above 5,000 feet before Madison and a descent. Even without the shortened stride of my stabbing Achilles, I would be exposed to lightning for several hours. Lightening rarely hits people. But when it does, it tends to hit young males, perhaps because they are the ones most likely to hike a ridge in a thunderstorm.

The rain let up. I made a dash for Mt Washington, it was only 1.5mi away and if the weather turned so could I. I climbed from slick rock to slick rock, landing flat footed with a short stride to avoid the sharp pain from my Achilles. My energy was high, bountiful really. The 20,000kcal in my backpack weighed only 6lbs, and I barely had any need to eat it. In a state of nutritional ketosis, my body was burning its own fat at such a high rate I could run up mountains.

At the top of Mt Washington, I was greeted fog so dense I could only see the gift shop from 20 feet away and the uncanny feeling of sticking my head out the window on the highway. The big ones always seem to have a gift shop...

I let gravity take me down.

Using my poles to unload my taped knees and landing flat-footed to unload my Achilles I raced the storm down the mountain.

It caught me before Mizpah Springs Hut.

In the hut I removed my shoes to check my feet. I stared at open sores on the back of each knuckle and toes so white and waterlogged I couldn't tell where the blisters began or ended. After a few spoonfuls of Thai cashew cream and a liter of water I checked the weather. For hours I was out in the wind and rain in only my shorts and the heat generated by hiking, now sitting here indoors and still soaked I was beginning to shiver. Tomorrow would be sunny. It was 4:30 and I had already covered 18miles, perhaps I could stay here tonight and do a big day tomorrow.

Was there any vacancy?

Yes, they had a room and warm shower.

I opened the door to check the weather and was met by a wall of water and a crack of thunder.

I'll stay.

It's $171.00 per night.

I'll go.

Out into the storm I ran, screaming like a banshee, stomping in puddles and pumping my arms wildly.

Relishing the fact that 75% of the energy of exercise is lost as heat. I needed every bit. I was soaked in adrenaline. The trees were not tall, but they were taller than me, which was enough. I sprinted through the clearings, pelted by hard bullets of rain. I went down more than once. Bleeding knuckles but no more. My pains receded and only the trail remained. The next place to put my foot was all that mattered. The trail got steeper and became a stream, then began a waterfall. Whitewater obscured my path. My pace slowed. I climbed down the ledges and grabbed the roots I had touched that morning. I began to shake. To go faster was to risk a fall and injury, to go slower was to risk a fall in body temperature. As the former would also lead to the later, I took my time and clenched my jaw against the cold.

I neared the Saco river and my Achilles reminded me of the abuse they had incurred thus far. I hoped my hasty packing had kept some of my warm gear dry.

It had not.

After 24 miles and 8, 177ft in 12hrs, I wrung out my soaked long underwear, hung my dripping hammock, pulled my damp down quilt over me. I listened to the beating of the rain on my shelter. I didn't sleep much that night.

White Mountains Day Three: July 2nd, 2017
After shuffling around my site like a Parkinsonian to avoid the bite of my Achilles, I decided to end the trip early. My ketogenic backpacking menu had given me all the energy I needed and then some. I felt like I had a turbocharged engine in a beat-up old pickup. No amount of engine tuning could compensate for the fact that the suspension was kaput.

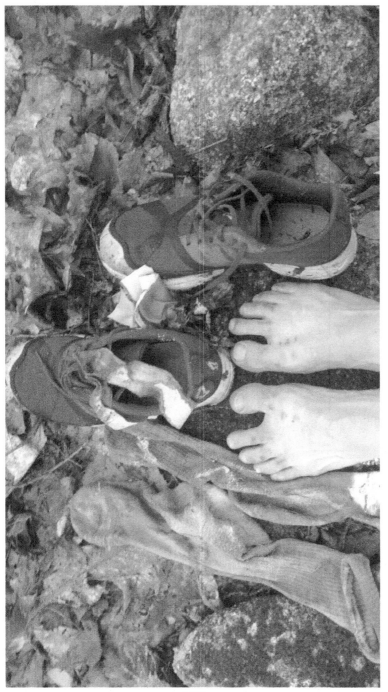

V: RECIPES

This section contains the recipes I created and perfected that fueled me with ketones on the Appalachian Trail. I hope you enjoy them as much as I have.

I have calculated the nutrition facts of each recipe by weight using either the ingredients' nutrition label or the http://myfitnesspal.com database for unlabeled items. I have assigned the following designations for each recipe according to the specific brands described in that recipe.

- p: Paleo. Free of grains, dairy, legumes, artificial colorings or preservatives. and minimally processed.
- v: Vegetarian
- g: Gluten free
- vegan: Free of all animal products

16. No Cook Recipes- Savory

Here you will find savory and satisfying combinations that
can be found in groceries stores along the trail or pre-
packed and mail dropped. The recipes range from fancy
hors d'oeuvres to trailer park snacks but each one packs at
least 1,000kcal and pairs a chewy or crunchy protein with
fat and a flavor counterpoint. To ensure a ketogenic effect,
don't get carried away with the protein. Taste, budget and
availability will determine when you go fancy and when
you just git er' done!

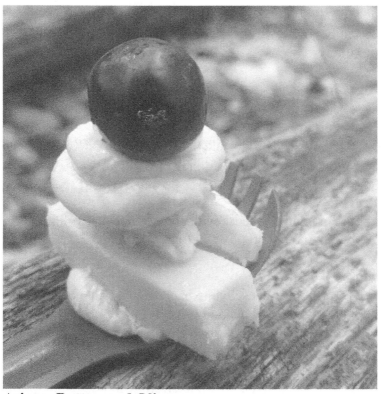

Asiago, Butter, and Olive v g

Prep: Simple
Wilder Ratio: 4.7
Cost/1000kcal: $4.68
Kcal/oz: 140

"Cheese, milk's leap towards immortality." -Clifton Fadiman

Hard cheeses get closer to immortality than any others. Having survived several years of aging they are hardy enough to survive a few days on the trail. The long shelf life of the hard cheeses is due to their low moisture and high salt content, exemplars of which are the Italian trio: Asiago, Parmesan, and Pecorino Romano. Asiago tends to

141

be the saltiest and pairing with brined Olives would certainly put it over the top if it weren't mellowed by a wad of butter.

Ingredients
- 4oz (113g) of Italian hard cheese. Asiago, Parmesan or Pecorino Romano.
- 8tbsp (4oz 113g) unsalted grass-fed butter (Kerrygold)
- 1 small (30g) pouch of black olives (Oloves)

Process
1. Pile a hunk of cheese with at least an equal volume of butter and put an olive on top.

Tips
- To preserve cheese while backpacking you need to keep it cool and dry. I accomplish this by keeping it buried deep in my backpack in its original packaging. In weather ranging from the 40-70 °F, I have kept cheese for weeks without issue. In 70-80 °F, it only lasts a few days... unless you are undeterred by mold.
- Pearls brand sells a convenient shelf stable plastic cup of olives. Olove brand as well as Trader Joe's sell convenient shelf stable pouches of olives.
- At home I like to pair these hard-Italian cheeses with a variety of antipastos such as sun-dried tomato, olive tapenade, pesto, marinated artichokes etc. Unfortunately, I haven't found shelf-stable, lightweight packaging for most of these antipastos (I haven't found an antipasto delicious enough to warrant the weight of packing a can or jar). You can bag an antipasto, but they don't last more than a day or so unless the weather is cold. If you find a lightweight prepackaged antipasto option, please let me know!

Asiago and Butter with Olives
Nutrition Facts

	(g)	(kcal)	(kcal %)
Fat	128	1152	91%
Carb	1	5	0%
Protein	26	103	8%
		1270	

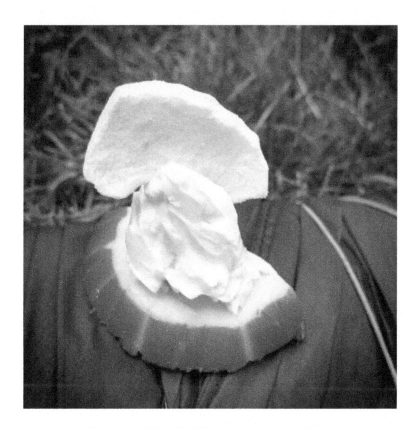

Smoked Gouda, Butter, and Apple v g

Prep: Simple
Wilder Ratio: 2.4
Cost/1000kcal: $3.38
Kcal/oz: 144

A smoky flavor wafts up from a background of soft butter and cheese and fills the palate until the crunch of apple releases a counterpoint of pome.

Ingredients
- 4oz (113g) of Smoked Gouda (Boar's Head)
- 8tbsp (4oz, 113g) unsalted grass-fed butter (Kerrygold)
- 1 pouch (10g) of freeze dried apples (Crispy Fruit)

Process

1. Cut a hunk of cheese, pile on at least an equal volume of butter and put an apple slice on top.

Tips

- The crispy freeze-dried apple provides crucial flavor and texture variety. If you are concerned about the sugar impairing fat burning, use less apple or switch to a less sweet fruit such as freeze-dried cranberries.
- To preserve cheese while backpacking you need to keep it cool and dry. I accomplish this by keeping it buried deep in my backpack in the original packaging. In weather ranging from the 40-70 °F, I have kept cheese for weeks without issue. In 70-80 °F, it only lasts a few days... unless you are undeterred by mold.

Smoked Gouda and Butter with Apples Nutrition Facts			
	(g)	(kcal)	(kcal %)
Fat	116	1044	84%
Carb	12	48	4%
Protein	36	144	12%
		1200	

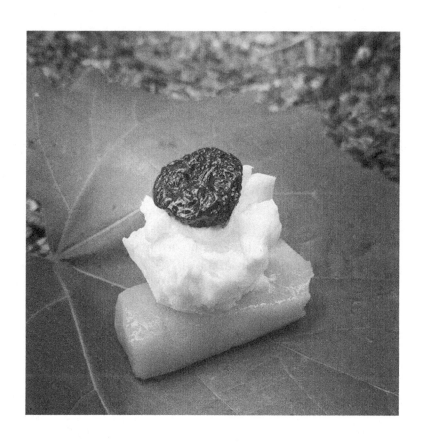

Cheddar, Butter, and Cherry v g

Prep: Simple
Wilder Ratio: 3.1
Cost/1000kcal: $2.75
Kcal/oz: 152

Cheddar and butter with a cherry on top. The cherry is a sweet and chewy barque on a golden sea.

Ingredients
- 4oz of Peppered Toscano (Trader Joe's)
- 8tbsp unsalted grass-fed butter (Kerrygold)

- 2.5tbsp (10g) cherries dried and unsweetened

Process
1. Cut a hunk of cheese, pile on at least an equal volume of butter and put a cherry on top.

Tips
- Cranberries are another good option if you can manage to find them unsweetened.

Cheddar, Butter, and Cherry Nutrition Facts			
	(g)	(kcal)	(kcal %)
Fat	124	1119	84%
Carb	11	43	4%
Protein	30	119	12%
		1270	

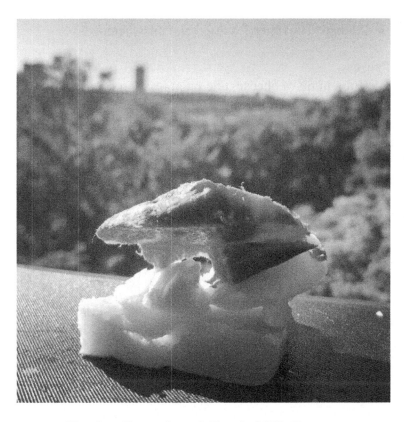

Chorizo, Roncal, and Goat's Milk Butter v

Prep: Simple
Wilder Ratio: 4.3
Cost/1000kcal: $5.70
Kcal/oz: 164

I crafted this combination while visiting the famous Zabar's epicurean grocery in NYC on a rest day during our Appalachian trail adventure. A delightfully complex gustatory journey ensued. The first taste to arrive is the goat butter which quickly melts away and allows the comforting sheep's milk Roncal to rise to the forefront only the be chased away by the rising dominance of spicy chorizo. Who says keto can't be gourmet, and on the trail at that! Furthermore, the high caloric density means that I ended up getting a pretty good deal as far as gourmet food goes. At least it beats caviar and marinated artichokes for price per 1,00kalby a wide margin!

Ingredients
- 1oz (28g) spicy cured chorizo (Palacio)
- 2oz (56g) Roncal (hard sheep's milk cheese)
- 3oz (6tbsp, 85g) salted goat's milk cheese

Process
1. Cut a thick slice of cheese, pile on at least an equal volume of butter and put a smaller piece of chorizo on top.

Tips
- To preserve cheese while backpacking you need to keep it cool and dry. I accomplish this by keeping it buried deep in my backpack in it's original packaging. In weather ranging from the 40-70 °F, I have kept cheese for weeks without issue. In 70-80 °F, it only lasts a few days... unless you are undeterred by mold.

Chorizo, Roncal, and Goat's Milk Butter Nutrition Facts			
	(g)	(kcal)	(kcal %)
Fat	98	884	91%
Carb	1	2	0%
Protein	22	90	9%
		985	

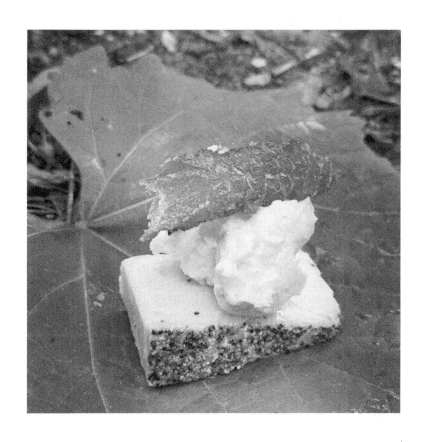

Toscano, Lard, and Salmon

Prep: Simple
Wilder Ratio: 3.7
Cost/1000kca/: $4.23
Kcal/oz: 169

Toscano cheese is nutty and sweet with enough black pepper to tie together land and sea. The lard introduces the guest but quickly exits to allow the smooth Toscano and chewy salmon to find they have sweetness in common. A leaf of miner's lettuce will provide the perfect touch of freshness if you can find it.

Ingredients
- 4oz (113g) of Peppered Toscano (Trader Joe's)
- 8tbsp (4oz, 113g) pastured lard (pastured Mangalitsa)
- 1oz 28g) (Salmon Jerky Bites (Epic)

Process
1. Cut a hunk of cheese, pile on at least an equal volume of lard and put a piece of salmon jerky on top.

Tips
- Finding a good salmon jerky can be tough. They either have too much added sugar or they taste terrible.
- Adding some bacon grease kicks this up a notch but if you are rendering yourself, make sure it is strained and completely free of water or it will go rancid.
- Romaine and butter lettuce are store bought replacements for the miner's lettuce if you happen to be in town. Plantain and dandelion leaf can also be used but are much more bitter.

Toscano, Lard, and Salmon Nutrition Facts			
	(g)	(kcal)	(kcal %)
Fat	144	1300	89%
Carb	2	8	1%
Protein	37	148	10%
		1460	

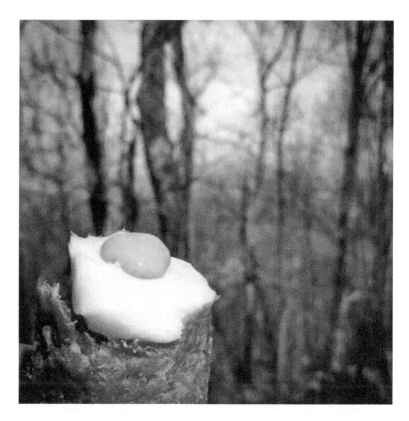

Salami, Lard, and Mustard

Prep: Simple
Wilder Ratio: 4.9
Cost/1000kcal: $2.85
Kcal/oz: 178

Dry salami is a backpacking classic. Shelf stable before opening, relatively calorie dense and absolutely delicious. Still, we can do better. The addition of lard brings salami squarely into the ketogenic circle. Yellow mustard plays a crucial role in brightening the palate and avoiding a savory overload.

Ingredients
- 4oz (113g) dry salami (Volpi)

- 8tbsp (4oz, 113g) lard (pastured Mangalitsa)
- 2 Mustard packets

Process
1. Cut a slice of salami, pile on as much lard as possible and finish with mustard on top.

Tips
- I have yet to find pastured pork salami.
- I have tried grey poupon, Sriracha and horseradish sauce but prefer yellow mustard to them all.

Salami, Lard, and Mustard Nutrition Facts			
	(g)	(kcal)	(kcal %)
Fat	138	1246	92%
Carb	0	0	0%
Protein	28	112	8%
		1360	

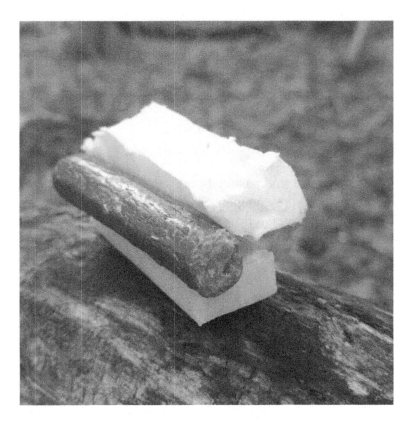

Pepperoni Swiss Rolls

Prep: Simple
Wilder Ratio: 3.2
Cost/1000kcal: $6.72
Kcal/oz: 152

Spicy pepperoni toned down by butter and sweetened by Swiss Emmental. Unlike the empty sugar loaded edible food-like-substance of the same name, this Swiss Roll delivers a ketogenic dose of meat, cheese and butter.

Ingredients
- 4 (92g) pepperoni sticks (Jack Link's) or slices.
- 4 (76g) Swiss cheese thin slices (Applegate Naturals)
- 8 tbsp (113g) grass fed unsalted butter (Kerrygold)

154

Process
1. Place two tablespoons of butter lengthwise on the cheese slice, place half the pepperoni stick on top and roll up.

Tips
- Dip in horseradish, mustard or Sriracha sauce for an extra kick.
- Stacking pepperoni slices, cheese and butter or laying slices side by side as in the picture is an equally tasty, albeit less novel option.

Pepperoni Swiss Rolls Nutrition Facts			
	(g)	(kcal)	(kcal %)
Fat	140	1260	88%
Carb	4	16	1%
Protein	40	160	11%
		1520	

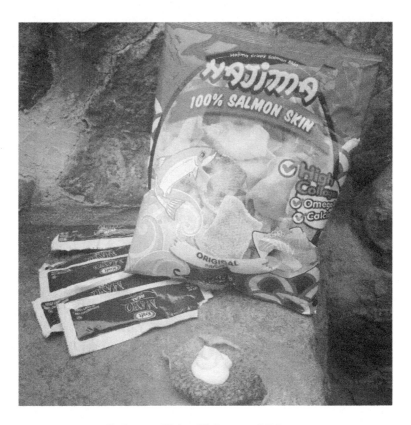

Salmon Skin Chips and Mayo

Prep: Simple
Wilder Ratio: 8.9
Cost/1000kcal: $5.83
Kcal/oz: 196

Fish skin chips are free of carbs and full of collagen. A keto food that has been hiding in the most unlikely place: beside the carb-laden snacks of your local Asian market. Dipped in mayo they are umami incarnate. This was one of my favorite foods on the Appalachian trail and I found myself ordering them on Amazon despite costing twice as much as at an Asian grocery. Unfortunately, I never saw an Asian grocery in any of the trail towns we stopped in

Ingredients
- 1 bag of salmon skins (20g)
- 124g of mayo, either 10 mayo packets (Kraft 12.4g each) or about 10 tablespoons.

Process
1. Dip your skins in mayo or squeeze mayo on top.

Tips
- The catch: I haven't found fish skin chips without msg.
- Mayo packets vs plastic tube? Many Asian grocers will carry the Japanese mayo brand Kewpie. This comes in a light-weight squeeze tube. It has a lighter, tangier flavor and has lasted me several days on the trail without spoiling, although some oil did separate out. The advantage of the packets is that you can eat just the amount you want without reducing the shelf life of the rest.
- Sir Kensington and Primal Kitchen both make delicious avocado mayonnaise that is light years healthier than standard mayo. But alas, I have not seen a trail friendly vessel for this superior mayo.

Salmon Skin Chips and Mayo Nutrition Facts			
	(g)	(kcal)	(kcal %)
Fat	107	963	98%
Carb	0	0	0%
Protein	12	24	2%
		1010	

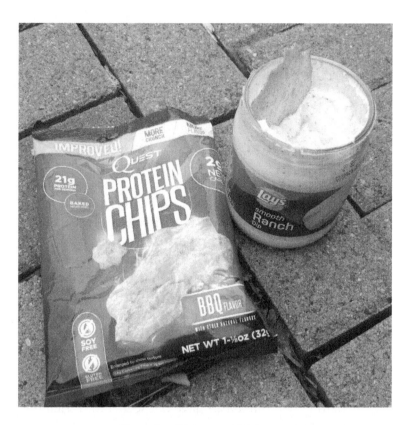

Protein Chips and Mayo g

Prep: Simple
Wilder Ratio: 4.2
Cost/1000kcal: $4.17
Kcal/oz: 185

We were 300 miles into our Appalachian Trail adventure and Jess was complaining about the lack of textural variety in our ketogenic backpacking food. Wandering down rabbit holes on Amazon with a weak data connection led to these chips being sent to our next mail drop. A brief experiment with ranch dip from the local drugstore was a failure, not enough fat, not shelf stable and not portable. Best to stick with mayo. Quest has removed the carbs and the frying but don't kid yourself, this is a processed food. If you are looking for some junk food without interrupting ketosis, look no further.

Ingredients
- 1 bag (32g) of protein chips (Quest)
- 124g of mayo, either 10 mayo packets (Kraft 12.4g each) or about 10 tablespoons.

Process
1. Dip your chips in mayo or squeeze mayo on top.

Tips
- Mayo packets vs plastic tube? The advantage of the packets is that you can eat just the amount you want without reducing the shelf life of the rest. The advantage of the tube is that it is cheaper... unless you get your packets for free.
- Sir Kensington and Primal Kitchen both make delicious avocado mayonnaise that is light years healthier than standard mayo. But alas, I have not seen a trail friendly vessel for this superior mayo.

Protein Chips and Mayo Nutrition Facts			
	(g)	(kcal)	(kcal %)
Fat	104	936	90%
Carb	4	16	2%
Protein	21	84	8%
		1030	

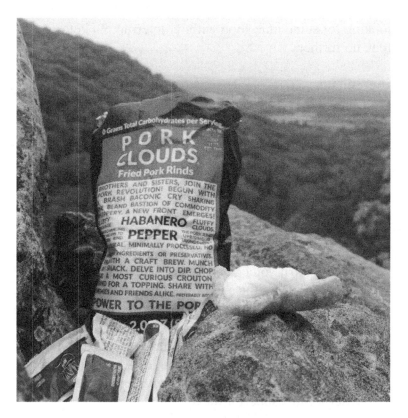

Hog Skins and Mayo g

Prep: Simple
Wilder Ratio: 6.1 (Bacon's Heir), 6.6 (Epic), 6.1 (4505), 8.0 (Galactic)
Cost/1000kcal: $3.86 (Bacon's Heir), $6.16 (Epic), $6.41 (4505), $5.45 (Galactic)
Kcal/oz: 195 (Bacon's Heir), 194 (Epic), 195 (4505), 195 (Galactic)

Hog skins, pork skins, pork clouds, pork rinds and chicharrones. The names and textures vary but they are all fried pork skin, a carb free crunchy snack that once symbolized unhealthy eating. It feels like cheating to know that this delicious combination is helping you burn fat.

Ingredients
- 1/2 bag of hog skins (30g) (Pork Clouds by Bacon's Heir, Pork Cracklings by Epic, Hog Skins by Galactic, or Chicharrones by 4505)
- 124g of mayo, either 10 mayo packets (Kraft 12.4g each) or about 10 tablespoons.

Process
1. Dip your hog skins in mayo or squeeze mayo on top.

Tips
- I strongly recommend pastured hog skins such as the Galactic brand. They are the healthiest and most sustainable as well as the tastiest. I have yet to come across them in a trail town.
- MSG and added sugar are common in hog skins, buying the plain version often avoids these additives.
- Mayo packets vs plastic tube? The advantage of the packets is that you can eat just the amount you want without reducing the shelf life of the rest. The advantage of the tube is that it is cheaper... unless you get your packets for free.
- Sir Kensington and Primal Kitchen both make delicious avocado mayonnaise that is light years healthier than standard mayo. But alas, I have not seen a trail friendly vessel for this superior mayo.

Galactic Hog Skins and Mayo Nutrition Facts			
	(g)	(kcal)	(kcal %)
Fat	112	1008	97%
Carb	0	0	0%
Protein	14	28	3%
		1060	

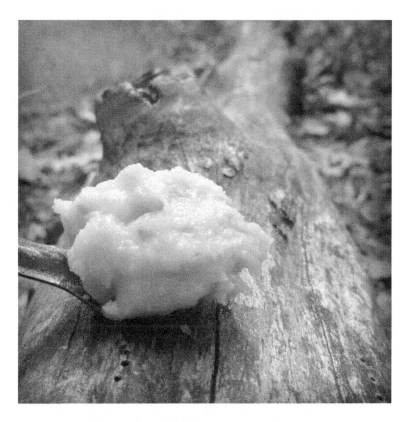

Seasoned Buffalo Ghee and Cashew Butter p v g vegan

Prep: Simple
Wilder Ratio: 4.1
Cost/1000kcal: $2.21
Kcal/oz: 212

A blend of savory spice, the butterscotch of ghee, and the sweetness of cashews all brightened to an exuberant yellow by inflammation fighting turmeric.

Ingredients

- 1 jar (8oz, 227g) seasoned Buffalo Ghee (Trader Joe's)
- 3/4c (192g) cashew butter (Trader Joe's)

Process
1. Mix together in a large well-sealing bag. Then double bag to prevent leaks.

Tips
- This is a better choice for cooler hikes. When the ghee is melted it becomes hard to eat.
- If you prefer a crunchier version, mix whole roasted cashews with ghee (pictured above).

Seasoned Buffalo Ghee and Cashew Butter Nutrition Facts			
	(g)	(kcal)	(kcal %)
Fat	316	2844	90%
Carb	54	216	7%
Protein	24	96	3%
		3120	

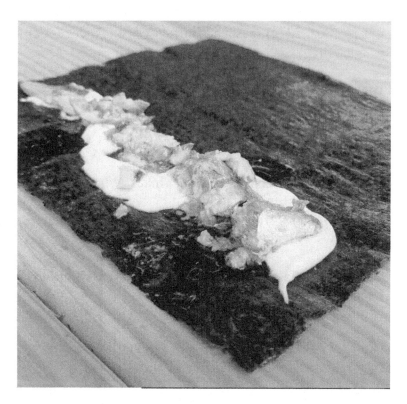

Nori Fish Wraps

Prep: Simple
Wilder Ratio: 5.4
Cost/1000kcal: $3.54
Kcal/oz: 130 (includes weight of pouch)

Every long-distance hiker knows that pouches of tuna are convenient sources of protein. But many hikers don't know that you can find more sustainable and healthier types of fish such as sardines and salmon in the same pouches. And even fewer know that if you drown your fish in mayo, wrap it in seaweed and sprinkle with lemon powder it becomes a delicious fat burning pack-lightening meal.

Ingredients

- 1 pouch (99g) sardines or salmon.
- 124g of mayo, either 10 mayo packets (Kraft 12.4g each) or about 10 tablespoons.
- 4 sushi nori wraps (Nagai)
- Assorted condiments: lemon packets, sriracha, soy sauce, wasabi, mustard, crunchy dried fish etc.

Process
1. Mix your fish and mayo in a bowl.
2. Spoon mixture onto nori and add condiments
3. Roll up and enjoy!

Tips
- Farmed fish is high in pro-inflammatory omega-6 fats and low in anti-inflammatory omega-3 and is harmful to the environment as well. Look for wild caught sustainably harvested fish with independent certifications to assure quality and accuracy such as Wild Alaska Pure, Better Seafood Bureau, and the Marine Stewardship Certificate.
- Mayo packets vs plastic tube? The advantage of the packets is that you can eat just the amount you want without reducing the shelf life of the rest. The advantage of the tube is that it is cheaper... unless you get your packets for free.
- Sir Kensington and Primal Kitchen both make delicious avocado mayonnaise that is light years healthier than standard mayo. But alas, I have not seen a trail friendly vessel for this superior mayo.
- These wraps can also be made with lard or coconut oil instead of mayo in cooler climates.

Nori Fish Wraps Nutrition Facts

	(g)	(kcal)	(kcal %)
Fat	108	972	92%
Carb	2	8	1%
Protein	18	72	7%
		1052	

17. No Cook Recipes- Sweet

These amazingly simple and delicious combinations can be made from ingredients found in grocery stores along the trail, or mixed ahead of time and shipped to mail drops. I recommend the latter method to secures a higher quality of ingredient for a better price.

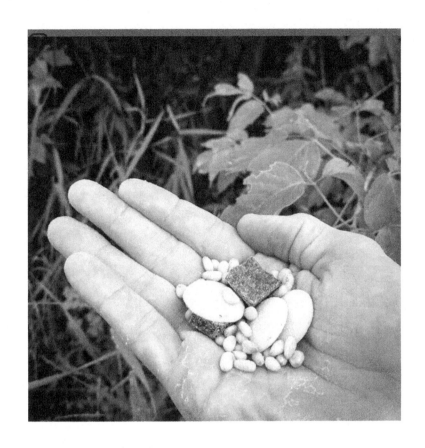

Dark Pine Trail Mix p v g vegan

Prep: Simple
Wilder Ratio: 4.9
Cost/1000kcal: $4.72
Kcal/oz: 198

Enter an opulent palace of chocolate and aromatic pine.
Sweet and fragrant pine nuts stand out alone on a dark
background of bitter chocolate, cocoa and cacao. A
scorching day on the trail transforms this trail mix into a
fudge fit for royalty.

Ingredients
- 1 cups (120g, 1/2 8oz bag) Pine nuts aka Pignolias (Trader Joe's)
- 1 bar (100g) Absolute Black Dark Chocolate with Cacao Nibs (Montezuma)
- 100g Cocoa butter wafers (Raw Organics)
- ½ tsp large salt flakes
- 1 tsp stevia powder

Process
1. Mix together in a large well-sealing bag.
2. Dust with salt and stevia powder to taste and shake.

Tips
- This mix tolerates higher temperatures than other trail mixes with chocolate.
- You can mix in walnuts, cashews, almonds or other nuts but I find this easily drowns out the pine nut flavor and reduced the Wilder ratio. Pine nuts are expensive, it's a travesty to put them in a mix and not taste them.

Dark Pine Trail Mix Nutrition Facts			
	(g)	(kcal)	(kcal %)
Fat	236	2124	92%
Carb	24	96	4%
Protein	24	96	4%
		2257	

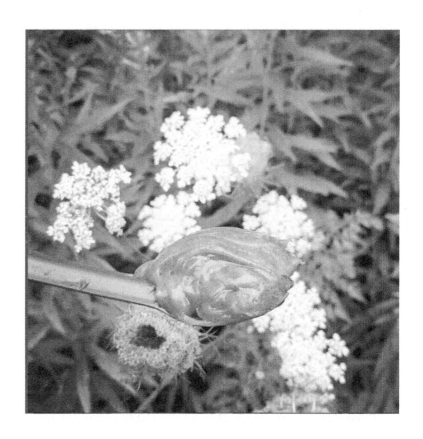

Buttered Nut Butter p v g

Prep: Simple
Wilder Ratio: 2.9 (peanut), 3.2 (cashew), 3.0 (almond)
Cost/1000kcal: $1.67 peanut, $2.55 cashew, $2.55 cashew
Kcal/oz: 183

Peanut butter's reputation as a high calorie, low cost, long
shelf life food has earned it a place in nearly every
backpack of America's long-distance trails. Peanut butter's
fancier friend, almond butter, is making more of an
appearance these days and thanks to Trader Joe's incredible
pricing, their luxurious acquaintance, cashew butter has
arrived on the scene. These three butters have similar

macronutrient ratios despite being completely unrelated botanically (peanuts are a legume, almonds are tree nuts and cashews are the seed of a drupe). Despite scoring higher than most standard backpacking fare on kcal/oz, these butters are too high in carbohydrates and protein to be ketogenic when eaten alone. The solution? Add more fat! Specifically, saturated fats that will maintain the thick consistency and pair well with the nutty flavor such as butter, coconut and palm oil. Mix and match nut butter and oils according to your taste and budget. Add a pinch of stevia powder if you are looking for something tasting more like Skippy. Some version of this quick and easy meal can be mixed up at any grocery store as well as some convenience stores and pharmacies.

Ingredients
- 1lb (454g) nut butter (Trader Joe's)
- 1lb (454g) grass-fed unsalted butter (Kerrygold) or coconut oil

Process
1. Stir butter into nut butter. If you only have one jar, add butter gradually as you eat. If you have two jars, divide the nut butter evenly, then mix in equal amounts of butter.

Tips
- Mix unsalted versions of both nut butter and butter and you might find the flavor a bit flat. Mix salted butter and unsalted nut butter for a mildly salt experience. Mix unsalted butter and salted nut butter for a saltier experience. Mix salted butter and salted nut butter for a dangerously salty experience.
- Mix in hot weather, enjoy in any weather.
- Grass fed butter will provide some healthy Omega-3 fatty acids.

- If using palm oil, make sure it comes from a rainforest safe source as the commercial palm oil industry is resulting in further deforestation.
- Coconut oil is higher in medium chain triglycerides which are easily turned into ketones and burned but not stored as fat. These MCTs provide immediate energy but may also cause indigestion in large quantities.
- If you store these mixes in bags, be sure to double bag to control leaks in hot weather.
- If you don't like the flavor of extra virgin coconut oil, use refined oil instead as it is nearly tasteless.

Peanut Butter and Butter Nutrition Facts			
	(g)	(kcal)	(kcal %)
Fat	576	5184	87%
Carb	98	392	7%
Protein	98	392	7%
		5860	

18. Homemade Recipes- Savory

A little work in the kitchen will yield delicious fuel you will look forward to on the trail. These recipes can be made at home in large batches that fuel many miles of hiking.

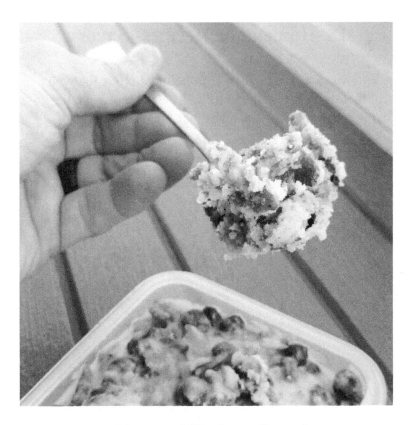

Bacon, Bison, and Blueberry Pemmican p g

Prep: Complex
Wilder Ratio: 6.3
Cost/1,000kcal: $8.20
Kcal/oz: 202

Pemmican is a mixture of dried meat and rendered fat that fueled American Indians during annual migrations and long hunting expeditions. It is the original American long-distance hiking food. Traditional recipes used bison, deer, elk and bear protein and fat in roughly equal ratios with dried berries being added seasonally. This is probably because fat was so hard to come by. I have increased the ratio to 75% fat and 25% protein for a more ketogenic effect. Bison tallow provides a solid and traditional

174

foundation for this pemmican, but freeze-dried blueberries add a textural twist and Applewood smoked bacon and drippings elevate this pemmican to a porcine Shangri-La.

Ingredients
- 1 jar (11oz, 311g) grass fed bison tallow (Epic)
- 2 packages (12oz, 340g) bacon (Niman Ranch)
- 1 bag (34g) freeze dried blueberries (Trader Joe's)

Process
1. Place bacon on two large backing pans and bake at 300 °F for 45min or until crispy but not burnt. Placing bacon on a raised grate in the pans results in drier bacon which is less likely to spoil.
2. Melt tallow gently with low heat then remove from heat.
3. Pour bacon drippings into tallow.
4. Cut bacon slices into strips or pieces with shears.
5. Stir all ingredients together.
6. Pour into a lock and lock container or a Ziploc or Mylar bag, then double bag.

Tips
- Freeze dried cranberries and cherries are other good alternatives.
- Dried fruit is also an option but does not provide the textural variety and still contains some water which increases the risk for spoilage.
- The more thoroughly you dry the bacon and render the drippings the longer the shelf life.
- You could use beef tallow and it would be closer to solid at room temperature, but it doesn't taste nearly as good.

Bacon, Bison, and Blueberry Pemmican Nutrition Facts

	(g)	(kcal)	(kcal %)
Fat	457	4111	96%
Carb	31	124	3%
Protein	17	170	2%
		4393	

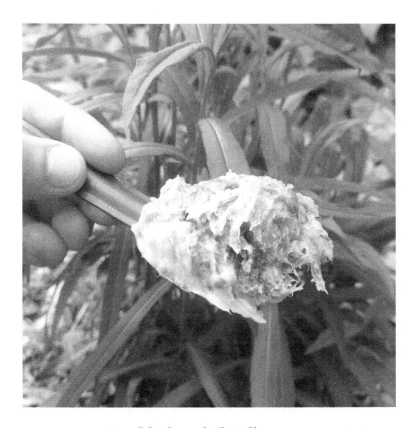

Machacado Lardican

Prep: Simple
Wilder Ratio: 4.2
Cost/1,000kcal: $4.12
Kcal/oz: 211

Pemmican is a mixture of dried meat and rendered fat that fueled American Indians during annual migrations and long hunting expeditions. It is the original American long-distance hiking food. Traditional recipes used bison, deer, elk and bear protein and fat in roughly equal ratios with dried berries being added seasonally. This is probably because fat was so hard to come by. I have increased the ratio to 75% fat and 25% protein by weight and use delicious pastured lard to create a ketogenic power fuel of outstanding flavor and function.

Ingredients
- 50g shredded dried beef aka Machacado (La Nortenita)
- 150g lard (pastured Mangalitsa)
- 1tbsp hickory liquid smoke (Colgin)

Process
1. Melt lard gently with low heat then remove from heat.
2. Stir in beef and smoke flavor
3. Pour into a Ziploc or Mylar bag and then double bag.

Tips
- Experiment with various spice combinations such as chili pepper, rosemary powder, Berber, and BBQ but use salt-free mixes because the shredded beef is already very salty.
- The quality of your lard will greatly influence the flavor. I recommend pasture-raised Mangalitsa lard.
- You could use beef tallow and it would be closer to solid at room temperature, but it doesn't taste nearly as good.

Machacado Lardican Nutrition Facts			
	(g)	(kcal)	(kcal %)
Fat	152	1368	91%
Carb	0	0	0%
Protein	36	143	9%
		1508	

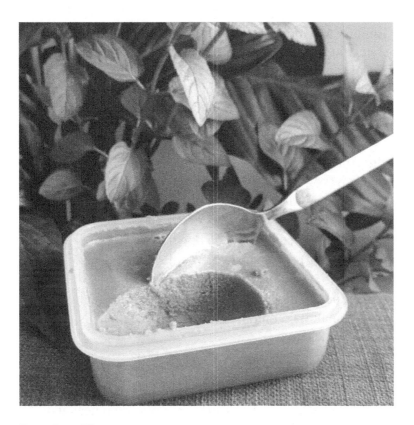

Beanless Hummus v g vegan
Prep: Complex
Wilder Ratio: 5.9
Cost/1,000kcal: $2.03
Kcal/oz: 216

In Israel, hummus is a hearty fast food meal served in a bowl with ground beef on top and pita on the side. I surmise that hummus started showing up in American supermarkets as a health food during the low-fat craze because in the process of crossing the Atlantic hummus somehow lost its high fat content and the remaining bland paste was dressed up in a bizarre array of spice costumes. This hummus recipe returns to the lipid laden roots of Israeli hummus, but snubs the beans altogether, instead

turning to the modern magic of molecular gastronomy and relying on mono and diglycerides to thicken
the oils to a paste. Essentially pure fat, this recipe creates enough breathing room in your macronutrient ratios to be served with wild onions, ground beef and perhaps even a low carb cracker!

Ingredients
- 4tbsp (64g) tahini paste (Trader Joe's)
- 1/16th tsp salt
- 1/8tsp garlic powder
- 1/4tsp citric acid or lemon powder
- 4tbsp (56g) extra virgin olive oil
- 4tbsp (56g) grapeseed or avocado oil
- 30g mono and diglycerides (Modernist Pantry)
- Optional: wild onions, ground beef, beef sticks, low carb crackers

Process
1. Immersion blend all ingredients over very low heat.
2. Once mixture reaches 140 °F, remove from heat and cool in refrigerator for at least 12 hours.
3. Dip grass fed beef sticks and green onion in hummus.

Tips
- High quality olive oil is the critical ingredient and should be the dominant flavor.
- If the olive oil is overwhelming, replace more of it with avocado or grapeseed oil. Avocado oil is the healthier option.

Beanless Hummus Nutrition Facts			
	(g)	(kcal)	(kcal %)
Fat	173	1554	93%
Carb	17	69	4%
Protein	12	48	3%
		1592	

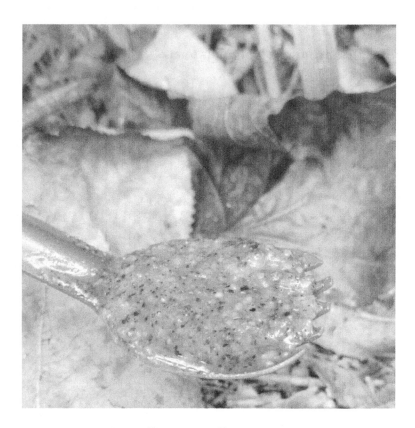

Parmesan Pesto v g

Prep: Moderate
Wilder Ratio: 3.8
Cost/1000kcal: $3.43
Kcal/oz: 191

An intense Italian medley of strong cheese, herbs and olive oil with the sweet overtones of pine nuts. This pesto is so good you may forget trying to find something to dip in it and just eat it by itself.

Ingredients
- 1/4c dried basil
- 1 cup (120g) pine nuts (Trader Joe's)
- ½ cup (60g) grated Parmesan cheese (Kraft)

182

- 1/4c (56g) extra virgin olive oil (Trader Joe's)
- 1/4c (56g) avocado oil (Baja Precious)
- 1/4tsp garlic powder

- Optional ~6 sprouted crackers (Livin Spoonful)

Process
1. Mix all ingredients then blend in food processor until smooth.

Tips
- If you use basil-infused oil instead of the avocado oil you can skip the step of adding basil, but you lose control over the amount of basil, the same is true for using garlic infused olive oil.
- Some may prefer more garlic, I start with a small amount and add slowly so as not to overwhelm the pine nuts.
- Adding dried kale, arugula and other greens adds additional nutrients. The Italian brand ROI makes a phenomenal arugula paste if you can find it.
- Macadamia nuts can be used instead of pine nuts, but the flavor will be much different.

Parmesan Pesto Nutrition Facts			
	(g)	(kcal)	(kcal %)
Fat	210	1890	89%
Carb	16	64	3%
Protein	40	160	8%
		2114	

19. Homemade Recipes- Sweet

These sweet but satisfying vegan recipes prove that a ketogenic diet doesn't have to include animals at all. This section includes a variety of nut butters and fudges that can be made relatively easily at home in large batches. A smooth and creamy texture is created by a combination of blended nuts and either saturated fats of liquid oils stabilized with mono and di-glycerides. The sweetness, intriguing flavors and vanishing caloric density of these recipes can entice you to consume a very large number of calories in a short period of time. Use this to your advantage if you were having trouble eating enough, otherwise eat slowly to give your brain time to let you know you are full.

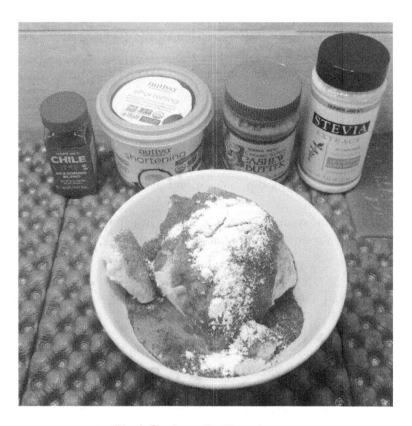

Thai Cashew Butter p v g vegan

Prep: Moderate
Wilder Ratio: 4.3
Cost/1,000kcal: $1.98
Kcal/oz: 214

This sweet and spicy cashew cream is an ultra-light backpacking superstar. A double batch yields 5,329kcal, weighs 1.5lbs and fits in a one-gallon bag. It maintains its consistency across a wide range of temperatures and can be eaten by the spoonful, added to coconut wraps or used as a dip.

Ingredients

- 2c (252g) lightly salted or Thai Chili Spiced cashews or cashew butter (Trader Joe's)
- 2tbsp chili-lime seasoning blend (Trader Joe's)
- 2tsp stevia powder (Trader Joe's)
- 2c (420g) blended sustainable palm and coconut oil shortening (Nutiva)

Process
1. Place nuts in food processor and blend.
2. Add stevia
3. Add chili spice if not using Thai Chili spiced cashews
4. Add shortening and blend until smooth

Tips
- Using Thai spiced cashews saves the step of adding spice but removes control over how spicy the butter will be.
- If you don't have a food processor you can mix the ingredients by hand, but it is best to soften the shortening with gentle heating first.

Thai Cashew Butter Nutrition Facts			
	(g)	(kcal)	(kcal %)
Fat	532	4784	91%
Carb	77	306	6%
Protein	47	187	4%
		5329	

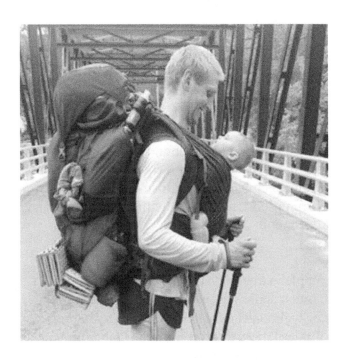

Smoky Apple Walnut Whip p v g vegan

Prep: Moderate
Wilder Ratio: 8.1
Cost/1,000kcal: $1.71
Kcal/oz: 232

Sustainable red palm and coconut oil create a decadent light cream that belies the high calorie content. Strong smoke and walnut flavors are balanced by notes of sweet apple in a delightfully enticing environment. Besides being delicious, this recipe is a ketogenic backpacking all-star: affordable and lightweight with a Wilder ratio off the charts.

Ingredients
- 2c (240g) walnuts
- 2c (420g) blended sustainable palm and coconut oil shortening (Nutiva)
- 1/4tsp apple extract
- 1/2tsp liquid smoke (Colgin)
- 1/4tsp salt
- 2tsp stevia powder (Trader Joe's)

Process
1. Place walnuts in food processor and blend.
2. Add a little palm and coconut oil shortening to prevent clumping and keep blending until smooth.
3. Add remaining shortening and all other ingredients and blend until smooth.

Tips
- Add the apple extract with care and mix thoroughly. A little too much apple with easily overwhelm the mix.
- You can use almonds instead of walnuts if you prefer but the Wilder ratio will drop from the higher protein and lower fat content of almonds.
- Using smoked almonds will save you the step of adding liquid smoke but will remove your control over how salty and smoky the cream becomes.

Smoky Apple Walnut Whip Nutrition Facts			
	(g)	(kcal)	(kcal %)
Fat	580	5220	95%
Carb	32	128	2%
Protein	40	160	3%
		5502	

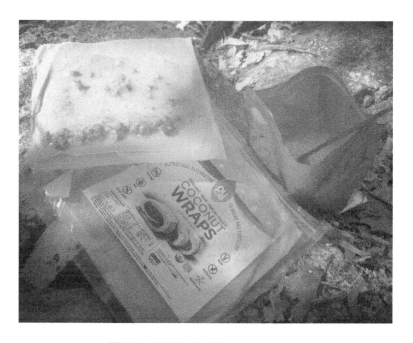

Walnut Maple Cream v g vegan

Prep: Complex
Wilder Ratio: 8.4
Cost/1,000kcal: $2.49
Kcal/oz: 221

Molecular gastronomy has pioneered the use many new ingredients in the kitchen, one of which is glycerin flakes. Glycerin flakes contains Mono and diglycerides which are derived from glycerin and fatty acids but do not contain any glycerin despite the name. These glycerides magically transform liquid oils to creams when mixed and cooled. This brings the delicious variety of nut oils into low carb free creams. While these nut oils can be eaten alone, their texture and flavor are richer, and their melting point is higher when blended with nut butters and saturated fats.

This walnut cream brings together two strong flavors of the North American woods: walnut and maple. The combination is a seductive dance of bitter and sweet.

Ingredients
- 1/2c (60g) walnut pieces pulsed or blended smooth (Trader Joe's)
- 1/2tsp stevia powder
- 1/2tsp maple flavoring
- 1/2tsp vanilla extract
- 1/8tsp salt
- 1/2c (112g) walnut oil (Spectrum)
- 30g glycerin flakes (Modernist Pantry)

Process
1. Mix all ingredients in a sauce pan.
2. Slowly heat to 140 °F.
3. Remove from heat and refrigerate for 12 hours uninterrupted.

Tips
- Add the maple extract with care and mix thoroughly. A little too much maple easily overwhelms the dish.
- Glycerin is technically a sugar alcohol that forms the backbone of triglycerides. It is probably absorbed and metabolized as a sugar when consumed alone, but its metabolism when bound to oils as in the recipe above is unclear. Despite this uncertainty I have tested very high blood ketone levels after eating 1,000kcal of oil set with glycerin flakes.

Walnut Maple Cream Nutrition Facts			
	(g)	(kcal)	(kcal %)
Fat	179	1608	95%
Carb	11	45	3%

Protein		10	40	2%
			1613	

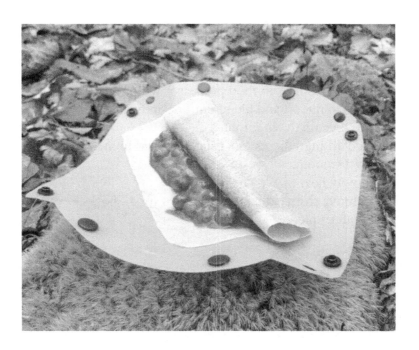

Chocolate Hazelnut Cream v g vegan

Prep: Complex
Wilder Ratio: 5.0
Cost/1,000kcal: $3.30
Kcal/oz: 206

Move over Nutella! This ketogenic chocolate hazelnut cream puts the sugared version to shame.

Ingredients
- 1/2c (112g) hazelnut oil roasted (La Tourangelle)
- 30g Glycerin flakes (Modernist Pantry)
- 1/2c (56g) hazelnuts roasted unsalted (Trader Joe's)
- 1/4c (20g) chocolate powder (Wild brand)

- 1tsp stevia powder (Trader Joe's)
- 1/8tsp salt

Process

Version 1: Creamy
1. Place hazelnuts in food processor with a small amount of hazelnut oil and blend until desired smoothness. This can take up to ten minutes.
2. Add all ingredients to a sauce pan and immersion blend until smooth.
3. Slowly heat to 140 °F.
4. Remove from heat and refrigerate for 12 hours uninterrupted.

Version 2: Crunchy
1. Whisk together all ingredients in a sauce pan.
2. Slowly heat to 140 °F.
3. Remove from heat and refrigerate for 12 hours uninterrupted.

Tips
- If you have an immersion blender you can use peanut butter. Without an immersion blender its best to use a powdered peanut butter as regular peanut butter is hard to mix evenly
- The same recipe can be used to make any combination of nut oil and nut butter. Almond butter with peanut oil is the best compromise of price and flavor I have found.

Chocolate Hazelnut Cream Facts			
	(g)	(kcal)	(kcal %)
Fat	177	1590	92%

Carb	23	93	5%
Protein	12	48	3%
		1621	

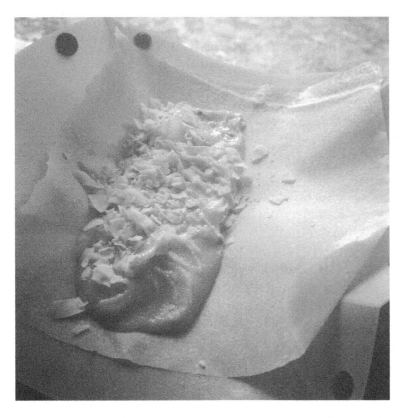

Peanut Cream with Cacao Nibs v g vegan

Prep: Complex
Wilder Ratio: 2.9
Cost/1,000kcal: $3.31
Kcal/oz: 199

A pure peanut lover's paradise with an occasional visiting cacao nib. This recipe transforms peanut butter to a ketogenic food but stays true to the peanut flavor by using peanut oil thickened with glycerin flakes instead of butter.

Ingredients
- 1/2c (112g) peanut oil (Snappy)
- 30g Glycerin flakes (Modernist Pantry)
- 1/2c (48g) peanut butter powder (P2B) OR peanut butter
- 1/4c (36g) cacao nibs (Navitas)
- 1tsp stevia powder (Trader Joe's)
- 1/8tsp salt

Process

Version 1: Peanut Butter Powder
1. Whisk together all ingredients in a sauce pan.
2. Slowly heat to 140 °F.
3. Remove from heat and refrigerate for 12 hours uninterrupted.

Version 2: Creamy Peanut Butter
1. Add all ingredients to a sauce pan and immersion blend until smooth.
2. Slowly heat to 140 °F.
3. Remove from heat and refrigerate for 12 hours uninterrupted.

Tips
- The same recipe can be used to make any combination of nut oil and nut butter. Almond butter with peanut oil is the best compromise of price and flavor I have found.

Peanut Cream with Cacao Nibs Nutrition Facts			
	(g)	(kcal)	(kcal %)
Fat	159	1428	87%
Carb	35	141	9%
Protein	20	80	5%
		1625	

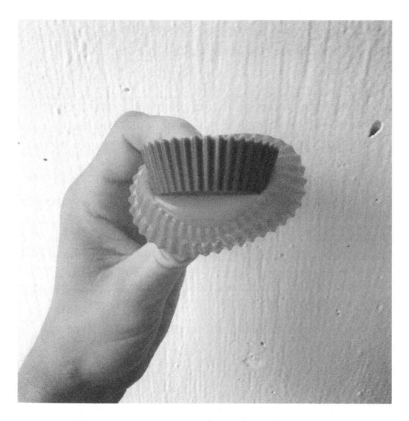

Green and Black's Almond Fudge p v vegan

Prep: Moderate
Wilder Ratio: 4.1
Cost/1,000kcal: $4.98
Kcal/oz: 213

Dark chocolate alone isn't dark enough. Take your chocolate beyond the dark side and into ketosis by adding cacao butter. A small amount of nut butter tames the bitter forces and makes a delicious keto super fuel. Stable through a wide range of temperatures, there's no excuse not to bring this chocolate on every adventure.

Ingredients

- 200g cocoa butter wafers (Raw Organics)
- 100g bar of Green and Black's 85%
- 50g creamy almond butter salted.

Process
1. Melt cacao wafers on low in microwave or stovetop.
2. Once wafers are melted, stir in chocolate bar until melted
3. Stir in nut butter.
4. Pour into bag or container and let sit to cool.

Tips
- The quality of the chocolate is key. If you don't like the chocolate by itself, you won't like the fudge. I have had great results from Green & Blacks Extra Dark and Lindt's 90%, with the latter being higher in carbs but easier to find
- If you don't use salted nut butter, add a 1/8tsp of salt

Green and Black's Almond Fudge Nutrition Facts			
	(g)	(kcal)	(kcal %)
Fat	278	2498	90%
Carb	46	184	7%
Protein	21	84	3%
		2661	

Montezuma Absolute Black Fudge _{p v vegan}

Prep: Moderate
Wilder Ratio: 4.8
Cost/1,000kcal: $3.98
Kcal/oz: 196

Darkest of the dark, Montezuma has inhabited the inhospitable land of 100% cacao. Take your chocolate beyond the dark side and into ketosis by adding cacao butter. A small amount of nut butter tames the bitter forces and makes a delicious keto super fuel. Stable through a wide range of temperatures, there's no excuse not to bring this chocolate on every adventure.

Ingredients
- 100g cacao wafers (Raw Organics)
- 100g absolute Black 100% Cacao with Nibs (Montezuma)c
- 50g creamy peanut or almond butter salted.

Process
1. Melt cacao wafers on low in microwave or stovetop.
2. Once wafers are melted, stir in chocolate bar until melted
3. Stir in nut butter.
4. Pour into bag or container and let sit to cool.

Tips
- The quality of the chocolate is key. If you don't like the chocolate by itself, you won't like the fudge. If using a sweeter brand such as Green & Blacks Extra Dark or Lindt's 90%, double the cacao wafers to 200g to ensure a ketogenic fudge.
- If you don't use salted nut butter, add a 1/8tsp of salt

Montezuma Absolute Black Fudge Nutrition Facts			
	(g)	(kcal)	(kcal %)
Fat	181	1629	91%
Carb	19	76	4%
Protein	19	76	4%
		1754	

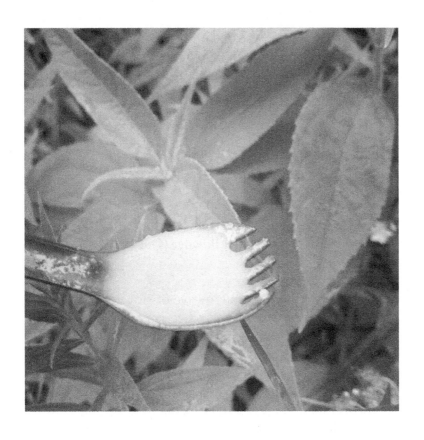

Pomegranate Macadamia Jetpack p v g vegan

Prep: Complex
Wilder Ratio: 4.9
Cost/1,000kcal: $4.12
Kcal/oz: 230

When you need energy right away, turn to medium chain triglycerides (MCT). MCTs enter the blood stream where they are used immediately as fuel. Coconut oil is rich in MCTs, up to 2/3 in some cases, but this recipe takes things above and beyond by adding MCT oil powder. Blended macadamia nuts and pomegranate team up to add a blast of antioxidants and incredible flavor.

Pomegranate Jetpack was one of the five foods I took on my two-day, 52-mile speed hike in the White Mountains of New Hampshire. A small amount goes a long way. I took one tablespoon twice a day.

Ingredients
- 2c (10oz, 283g) macadamia nuts roasted and lightly salted (Trader Joe's)
- 1/2c (112g) strained coconut oil (Trader Joe's)
- 2tbsp (15g) pomegranate powder (Nutiva)
- 8 scoops (72g) MCT Oil Powder (Quest)

Process
1. Soften coconut oil in microwave or stovetop.
2. Add all ingredients to food processor and blend.
3. Pour into a tightly sealing plastic jar (fills one reused 16oz nut butter jar)

Tips
- Pomegranate powder can be exchanged for other low-carb superfruit powders such as baobob or maqui powder or omitted altogether.
- This recipe uses MCT oil powder instead of oil because the powder form provides a better consistency and is less likely to cause digestive upset. I recommend using a MCT oil powder with a pre-biotic carrier such as corn starch.
- If you don't use salted macadamias, add a 1/8tsp of salt, but you must add the salt to the nuts and blend alone first, if you try to add it at the end it won't mix well because salt doesn't dissolve in oil.

Pomegranate Macadamia Jetpack Nutrition Facts			
	(g)	(kcal)	(kcal %)
Fat	386	3472	92%
Carb	60	239	6%
Protein	19	76	2%
		3663	

20. Trailmade Recipes- Savory

The value of a hot meal increases exponential with the number of cold wet days on the trail. Those who eschew the trail cooked meal because of the weight of stove, fuel and cookware, often find themselves pushing for extra miles to get a hot meal in town. Fortunately, backcountry cooking technology has become more reliable and lighter and now a hot meal can be made in five minutes for the price of carrying an additional 22 ounces. The recipes in this section consist primarily of soups and hot beverages which only require hot water. This saves time both cooking and cleaning and means you can enjoy a hot meal anytime. The servings sizes for these meals range around 1,000kcal, and represent my palatable upper limit for fat content. If you need fewer calories, you can either make a smaller batch, add more water or reduce the fat quantity.

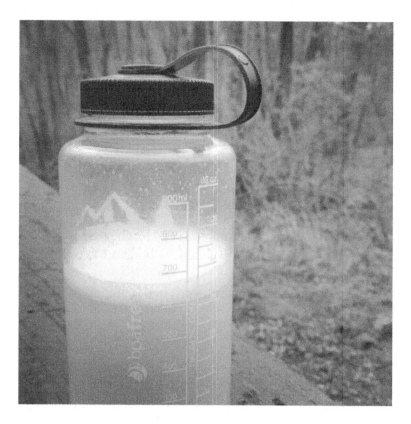

Buttered Broth p

Prep: Simple
Wilder Ratio: 14.8 (Orrington), 6.8 (Lonolife), 6.1 (Protein Essentials)
Cost/1000kcal: $2.42 (Orrington), $4.42 (Lonolife), $4.10 (Protein Essentials)
Kcal/oz: 185 (Orrington), 186 (Lonolife), 186 (Protein Essentials)

A bottle of hot buttered broth makes donning your wet socks and shoes a little easier. The simple combination of butter and bullion is quick to prepare even with stiff chilly fingers and a half-sleeping brain. Using a high-quality bone broth base provides essential amino acids and cartilage supporting proteoglycans. Grass fed butter vides anti-inflammatory omega-3 fatty acids and 15% quick burning medium chain triglycerides. A variety of high quality bullion and broth packets will keep you looking forward to the next morning. Using cheap bullion instead of bone broth and corn-fed instead of grass-fed butter would make this a very affordable breakfast. Just don't expect the same flavor or health benefits. Ingredients matter!

Ingredients
- 3 cups (700ml) hot water
- 1 bouillon cube or scoop/packet of broth powder (12-18g). (Orrington bullion, Lonolife bone broth or Protein Essentials bone broth)
- 8tbsp (4oz, 112g) unsalted grass-fed butter (Kerrygold)

Process
1. Begin heating water.
2. Place butter and bullion or broth scoop/packet in a heat tolerant thermos or water bottle such as a Nalgene.
3. When water has reached desired temperature, pour into bottle and shake.
4. Wait 1min then loosen seal carefully to release pressure.

Tips
- Be sure to use unsalted butter to avoid an over-salted experience.
- If you are starting with clean water, you can save fuel by only heating the water up to the desired temperature. I heat mine to the point where I can't stick my finger in it for more than three seconds. If it's a cold day and I plan on hiking with my broth I will heat the water more.
- Adjust the concentration of bullion or bone broth and butter according to your preferences and caloric needs.

Buttered Broth (Protein Essentials) Nutrition Facts			
	(g)	(kcal)	(kcal %)
Fat	88	794	93%
Carb	3	10	1%
Protein	12	48	6%
		865	

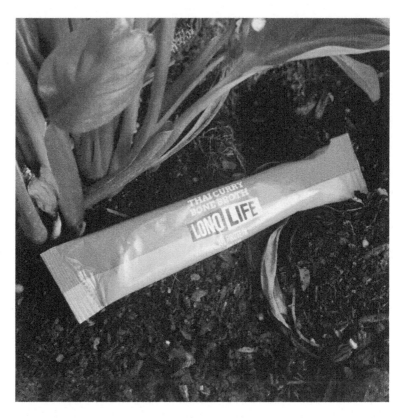

Thai Beef Bone Broth p g

Prep: Moderate
Wilder Ratio: 6.5
Cost/1000kcal: $5.41
Kcal/oz: 232

This savory beverage is a welcome antidote to cold dreary
weather at any time of day or night. Coconut oil provides
60% immediately usable medium chain triglycerides, the
tallow provides a hearty flavor and the bone broth base
provides essential amino acids and cartilage supporting
proteoglycans. Lonolife brand bone broth and Epic brand
grass-fed tallow make this nourishing broth a bit pricey.

One could make a cheaper albeit less nutritious broth with Thai curry spice paste and coconut oil.

Ingredients
- 3 cups (700ml) hot water
- 1 stick packet (16g) of Thai curry beef bone broth (LonoLife)
- 3tbsp (42g) beef tallow grass-fed (Epic brand)
- 3tbsp (42g) extra virgin coconut oil (Nature's Way)
- Optional: 1tsp (5g) soy lecithin for emulsification. Either liquid (Fearn) or powdered (Modernist Pantry)

Process
1. Begin heating water.
2. Place tallow, coconut oil and broth packet in a heat tolerant thermos or water bottle such as a Nalgene.
3. When water has reached near boiling, pour into thermos and shake.
4. Wait 1 minute, then loosen seal carefully to release pressure.

Tips
- Because of the high saturated fat content of tallow and coconut oil, the water will need to be hot to melt it. In cool weather I boil the water first, then wait a few minutes after mixing until it is cool enough to drink.
- Be sure to drink it while still warm, once it cools down the oil clumps and separates and the palatability of then broth plummets.
- Adjust the concentration of broth powder and the ratio of tallow to coconut oil to your taste and calorie needs. Adding a teaspoon of peanut oil further enhances the complexity of the flavor.
- Use refined coconut oil if you don't like the taste of coconut.

Thai Beef Bone Broth Nutrition Facts

	(g)	(kcal)	(kcal %)
Fat	84	756	94%
Carb	3	12	1%
Protein	10	40	5%
		828	

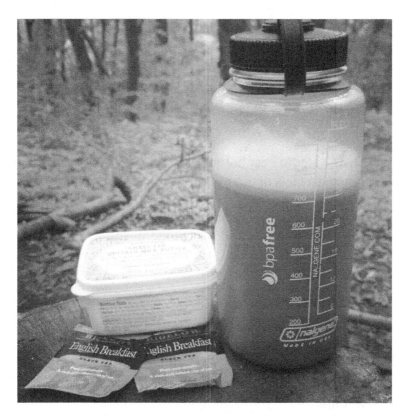

Black Tea with Buffalo Butter p v g

Prep: Moderate
Wilder Ratio: Zero carbs and protein
Cost/1000kcal: $1.88
Kcal/oz: 206

This recipe was inspired by Tibetan yak butter tea which I
have never tasted but is rumored to be energizing but not
appetizing. The arrival of water buffalo butter in Trader
Joe's brought a less buttery and more gamey flavor that
complements the black tea without overwhelming it.
Starting your day with this buttered tea free of carbs and
protein is essentially a fat fast, giving you the benefits of
fasting such as autophagy without the hunger or energy dip.

Ingredients
- 3 cups (700ml) hot water
- 2 bags of black tea (Newman's Own Organic)
- 8tbsp (40z, 112g) grass fed buffalo butter (Trader Joe's)

Process
1. Heat water to near boiling
2. Place tea bags in thermos or heat tolerant water bottle such as a Nalgene.
3. Leave tea to steep for 6min then remove tea bags.
4. Add buffalo butter and shake vigorously.
5. Wait 1min then loosen seal carefully to release pressure.

Tips
- Adjust the duration of steeping and the amount of butter to your taste preference and energy needs.
- If you are starting with clean water, you can save fuel and time by just heating the water up just shy of boiling.

Black Tea and Buffalo Butter Nutrition Facts			
	(g)	(kcal)	(kcal %)
Fat	96	864	100%
Carb	0	0	0%
Protein	0	0	0%
		864	

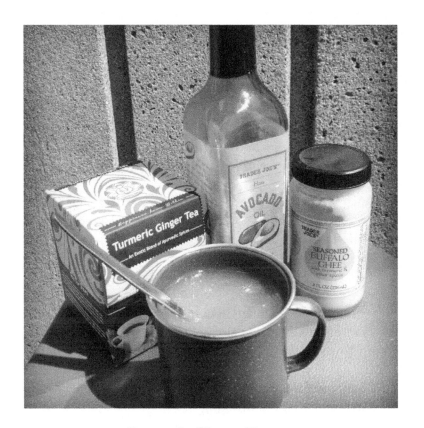

Turmeric Ginger Tea p v g

Prep: Complex
Wilder Ratio: zero carbs and protein
Cost/1,000kcal: $2.43
Kcal/oz: 230

Harness the anti-inflammatory powers of turmeric with this healing tea. A blend of spice and buffalo ghee engage the senses and transports you to distant lands.

Ingredients
- 3 cups (700ml) hot water
- 3bags of turmeric ginger tea (Buddha Teas)
- 4 tbsp (2oz, 60g) spiced buffalo ghee with turmeric (Trader Joe's

- 4 tbsp (2oz, 56g) avocado oil (Baja Precious)
- Optional: 1tsp (5g) soy lecithin. Either liquid (Fearn) or powdered (Modernist Pantry)

Process
1. Begin heating water.
2. When water nears boiling, turn off heat and place tea bags in water. Steep for 6min, longer for stronger flavor.
3. When tea is done steeping, remove bags and pour tea into Nalgene with butter, avocado oil and lecithin.
4. Seal and shake to mix.
5. Wait for pressure to settle before opening.

Tips
- Grass fed buffalo ghee with turmeric is now sold at Trader Joe's in a convenient 8oz bottle that is relatively light, is shelf stable and will make four servings of this tea.
- If you forego the lecithin, you will need to shake periodically before drinking
- If you are starting with clean water, you can save water and fuel and reduce the risk of burning yourself by heating the water only up to the desired temperature.

Turmeric Ginger Tea Nutrition Facts			
	(g)	(kcal)	(kcal %)
Fat	120	1077	100%
Carb			0%
Protein			0%
		1077	

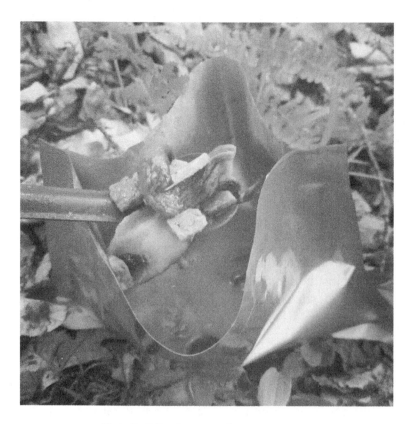

Triple Mushroom Soup p v g vegan

Prep: Complex
Wilder Ratio: 10.5
Cost/1000kcal: $3.17 (All ingredients purchased on Amazon.com)
kCal/oz: 221

This blend of mushrooms has a savory taste and aroma that complements an evening in nature. Each type of mushroom brings it's own variation on a sylvan theme.

Ingredients
- 500ml hot water
- 5g white mushrooms (dried)
- 5g oyster mushrooms (dried)

213

- 5g shitake mushrooms (dried)
- 1/3 cube vegetable bullion
- 1 bay leaf
- 10 rosemary leaves or 1/4tsp rosemary powder
- 1/8tsp salt
- 1/8tsp pepper
- 1tsp (5g) liquid soy lecithin (Fearn)
- 1/2c (112g) neutral oil such as avocado or grapeseed

Process
1. Heat water to boiling.
2. Place all ingredients except oil in heat tolerant bowl or bottle such as a Nalgene.
3. Add just boiled water, stir and let sit for ten minutes.
4. Add oil, stir and enjoy.

Tips
- I have packed all the ingredients including the oil together in one heat-sealed Mylar bag. This made packing more convenient as I didn't have to match the dry ingredients with their respective oil. However, the oil coated mushrooms and slowed the rehydration process.
- Adjust the amount and types of mushrooms according to your carb tolerance and taste preferences.
- Most of the dried mushrooms that I bought had widely varying or absent nutrition facts, so I used values from MyFitnessPal which should be treated with some suspicion.

Triple Mushroom Soup Nutrition Facts			
	(g)	(kcal)	(kcal %)
Fat	117	1052	96%
Carb	7	27	2%
Protein	4	17	2%

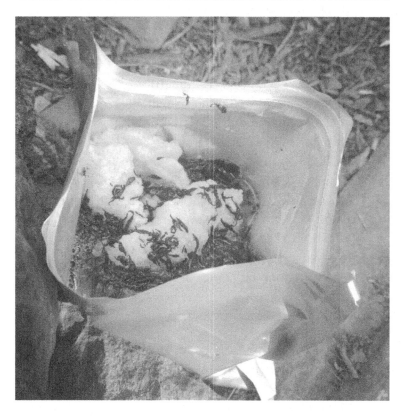

Seaweed Maw Soup p g

Prep: Complex
Wilder Ratio: 3.2
Cost/1000kcal: $6.81
Kcal/oz: 191

Enjoy a taste of the ocean in the backcountry. Dulce brings notes of tea, wakame brings sweetness, while nori and fish maw bring umami. Choosing duck fat adds a rich flavor while choosing avocado oil leaves the seaweed on center stage. Bright notes of ginger and black pepper balance the hearty umami and salty anchovies. Your only carbs are the seaweed and seasoning, so you can bump up the flavor and texture of the soup by adding more of these if you know you can stay in ketosis on more carbs.

Ingredients

- 500ml hot water
- 5g dulse seaweed dried (Rahimali)
- 5g sushi nori seaweed dried (Nagai)
- 5g wakame seaweed dried (VitaminSea)
- 5g kombu seaweed dried (Rahimali)
- 5g puffed fish maw dried
- 10g anchovies dried
- 1/2tsp sesame ginger vegetable seasoning (Simply Organic)
- 10g bonito flakes
- 1/4tsp black pepper
- 1/2c (112g) duck fat (Epic) or avocado oil (Baja Precious)

Process

1. Begin heating water.
2. Place all ingredients except oil in a bowl or heat tolerant bottle such as a Nalgene.
3. Add boiled water.
4. Stir and let sit for 10min.
5. Add duck fat or avocado oil, stir and enjoy.

Tips

- I have packed all the ingredients including the oil together in one heat-sealed Mylar bag. This made packing more convenient as I didn't have to match the dry ingredients with their respective oil and it didn't seem to hinder the rehydration.
- I have included a wide variety of seaweed in this recipe but often I make each meal a little different by adding only a few different types of seaweed.

- I have noticed a big difference in hydration times for different brands of kelp. Some become soft and easy to chew while others remain like rawhide.
- Most of the seaweed I bought did not have nutrition labels, so I used the values for nori for the entire weight of seaweed in the recipe.
- The high cost of this meal is based on ordering seaweed and fish maw on Amazon as well as using pastured duck or avocado oil. Buy your dry ingredients at the local Asian market and use canola oil and this becomes an affordable meal.
- The fish maw adds a mild but distinct taste to the dish. When rehydrated in the soup it takes on a soggy texture while still being hard to chew. You may prefer to eat the fish maw dry like a cracker or exclude it altogether.

Seaweed Maw Soup Nutrition Facts			
	(g)	(kcal)	(kcal %)
Fat	116	1046	88%
Carb	12	47	4%
Protein	25	100	8%
		1194	

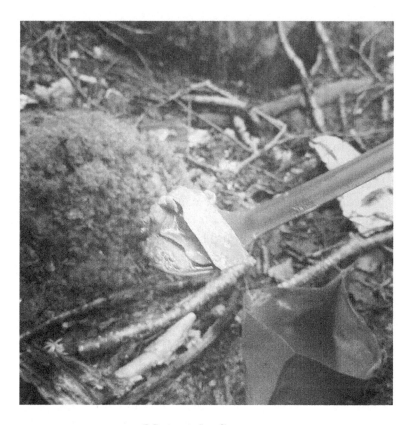

Matsutake Soup p g

Prep: Complex
Wilder Ratio: 8.4
Cost/1000kcal: $8.19
Kcal/oz: 216

The traditional dashi broth is made from flakes of dried red fin tuna and kelp. The nutty, coniferous, aromatic flavor of the matsutake is the star of the show and the avocado oil does its best to hide in the background while providing the necessary calories. Store bought dried matsutake mushrooms are safe but pricey, but if you have the skills to forage wild matsutake, the experience is unparalleled.

Ingredients
- 500ml hot water
- 5g kombu kelp (Rahimali)
- 5g bonito flakes
- 2 tsp liquid aminos (Braggs)
- ¼ tsp salt
- 10g dried matsutaki (Amazon)
- ½ c (112g) avocado oil (Baja Precious)

Process
1. Begin heating water.
2. Place all ingredients except oil in a bowl or heat tolerant bottle such as a Nalgene.
3. Add boiled water.
4. Stir and let sit for 10min.
5. Add oil, stir and enjoy

Tips
- Matsutakes are expensive because they grow symbiotically with pine and oak tree roots and only fruit sporadically making cultivation difficult and leaving foraging as the primary source. I once found a deal on dried Matsutakes at my local grocery co-op for $65/lb. Prime fresh Matsutake mushrooms sell for hundreds of dollars in Japan. Luckily you only need an ounce for this recipe and you won't regret it.

Matsutake Soup Nutrition Facts			
	(g)	(kcal)	(kcal %)
Fat	115	1038	95%
Carb	7	30	3%
Protein	6	25	2%
		1093	

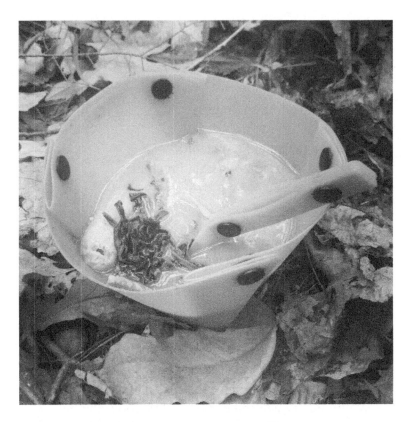

Spicy Sesame Mushroom Soup p g

Prep: Complex
Wilder Ratio: 3
Cost/1000kcal: $5.93
Kcal/oz: 217

Wood ear mushrooms are exactly the kind of fantastical ingredient you might expect in a fairy tale soup. This soup brings flavors that are far from familiar to most western audiences. The novelty and intrigue banishes mealtime boredom and transports you to another world no matter how close or far from home you happen to be.

Ingredients

220

- 500ml hot water
- 20g wood ear fungus shredded and dried
- 5g of oyster mushroom
- 1tbsp sesame ginger vegetable seasoning (Simply Organic) (or 1/8tsp ginger)
- 1/4 tsp Japanese 7 spice (spicy)
- 1tsp(5g) soy lecithin
- 1/4c (56g) duck fat or avocado oil
- 2tbsp (28g) toasted sesame oil

Process
3. Begin heating water.
4. Place all ingredients except oil in a bowl or heat tolerant bottle such as a Nalgene.
5. Add boiled water.
6. Stir and let sit for 10min.
7. Add oil, stir and enjoy

Tips
- You can mix and match ingredients with the seaweed stomach soup for variety.
- To speed up the softening of the wood ear mushrooms you can add them to the water as you heat it.
- If you are feeling adventurous, add bamboo fungus. But be careful, its strong flavor easily dominates the soup and its soggy slimy texture is unlike most western foods.
- The high price of this meal is calculated from the price of dried fungus on Amazon and pastured duck fat. Buy your dried mushrooms at the local Asian market and substitute for a lower quality duck fat or replace avocado oil with canola oil and you will spend a lot less.

Spicy Sesame Mushroom Soup Nutrition Facts			
	(g)	(kcal)	(kcal %)
Fat	116	1046	88%
Carb	12	47	4%
Protein	25	100	8%
		1194	

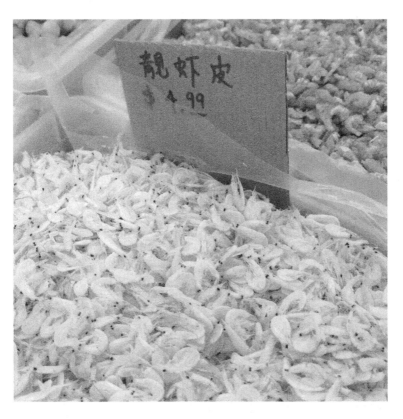

Thai Hot and Sour Soup (Tom Yum) p

Preparation: Complex
Wilder Ratio: 4.2
$/1000kcal: $3.16
Kcal/oz: 207

I didn't grow up with spicy food and I would tear up with
the most minor of spicy encounters such as a jalapeno in
jack cheese. In my late 20s, I decided to improve my spicy
food tolerance during the two months leading up to a trip to
Thailand. I started by sprinkling chili powder on
everything, just a little at first, then more and more. I
worked my way up from eating poblanos to jalapenos and
finally habanero. Each week I added a few more Thai
birds-eye chilis to my meals. Tears were shed, water was

guzzled, and on more than one occasion I was heard running around the house alternately screaming and sucking on ice and mint. My goal was met when I sat down at a night market in Chang Mai and ate a whole bowl of a hot and sour seafood soup known as Tom Yum. A handful of dried birds-eye chilis make for cheap entertainment on a thru hike. Just start slow and add one chili at a time as ice and mint aren't always at hand in the backcountry.

Ingredients
- 500ml hot water
- 1/3 packet (25g) Tom Yum soup powder (East Kitchen)
- 20g dried tiny glass shrimp
- 1tsp (5g) soy lecithin for emulsification. Either liquid (Fearn) or powdered (Modernist Pantry)
- 1/4c (56g) extra virgin coconut oil (Nature's Way)
- 1/4c (56g) avocado oil (Baja Precious)
- Optional: dried Thai birds eye chilis to taste
- Optional: 10g dried white mushrooms
- Optional: 2 dried kaffir lime leaves
- Optional: 2 dried galangal leaves
- Optional: 2 dried lemongrass leaves

Process
1. Mix the Tom Yum paste, shrimp and mushrooms in the water as you heat it.
2. Pour in the lecithin slowly while stirring.
3. Remove from heat.
4. Remove the stems, rip up the leaves and toss in the kaffir lime, galangal and lemongrass
5. Stir in the avocado and coconut oil slowly

Tips:
- Getting pastes and powders to dissolve and blend smoothly on the trail can be difficult. One strategy is to pour all the ingredients into a Nalgene bottle then add

an agitator such as a short mini spoon or a few small clean pebbles then shake.

- If the Tom Yum paste is already too spicy for you, increase the water or decrease the paste.
- If you want more texture and can handle the saltiness, add more shrimp.
- If you need more calories, keep adding fat until you get to the upper limit of palatability or digestibility. A ¼c of coconut oil is my safe upper limit, I have consumed ½c on several occasions only to have a stomach ache and vomit several hours later.
- If you need a longer shelf life or don't like the coconut flavor, use refined coconut oil.
- If the weather is cool you will need to bring the water up to boiling to melt the coconut oil.
- When shopping for Tom Yum paste, look carefully at the carbs and serving size, many Tom Yum pastes are high in sugar.

Thai Hot and Sour Soup (Tom Yum) Nutrition Facts			
	(g)	(kcal)	(kcal %)
Fat	120	1082	91%
Carb	14	57	5%
Protein	14	56	5%
		1195	

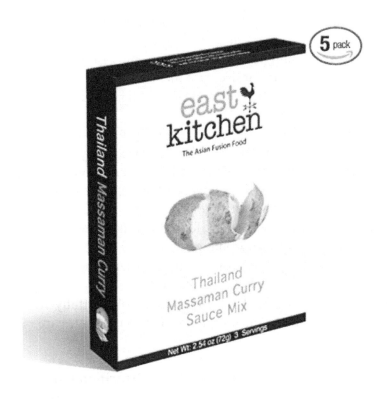

5 pack

Thailand Massaman Curry

east kitchen
The Asian Fusion Food

Thailand
Massaman Curry
Sauce Mix

Net Wt: 2.54 oz (72g) 3 Servings

Massaman Chicken Curry

Prep: Complex
Wilder Ratio: 3.8
Cost/1000kcal: $3.72
Kcal/oz: 213

Massaman curry is a staple of Thai cuisine said to be brought to the Thai court of Ayutthaya by a Persian Silk Merchant. You can keep things simple with the curry powder, coconut oil and chicken or embellish with peanut butter, cashews and dried onion.

Ingredients
- 500ml hot water

- 20g dehydrated chicken (Valley Food Storage)
- 1/3 packet (25g) Massaman chicken powder (East Kitchen)
- 10g Fried onion
- 1tsp (5g) soy lecithin. Either liquid (Fearn) or powdered (Modernist Pantry)
- 3 tbsp (42g) coconut oil extra virgin coconut oil (Nature's Way)
- 3 tbsp (42g) peanut oil (Snappy)
- 1/4c (56g) avocado oil (Baja Precious)
- Optional: 1tbsp peanut butter

Process
1. Mix the chicken and Massaman curry paste or powder in the water as you heat it, stirring to insure it dissolves.
2. Pour in the lecithin slowly while stirring.
3. Remove from heat.
4. Stir in the avocado and coconut oil.
5. Sprinkle fried onions on top

Tips:
- Getting pastes and powders to dissolve and blend smoothly on the trail can be difficult. One strategy is to pour all the ingredients into a Nalgene bottle then add an agitator such as a short mini spoon or a few small clean pebbles then shake.
- If you want more texture and can handle the protein, add more chicken.
- If you need more calories, keep adding fat until you get to the upper limit of palatability or digestibility. A ¼c of coconut oil is my safe upper limit, I have consumed ½ on several occasions only to have a stomachache and vomit hours later.
- If you need a longer shelf life or don't like the coconut flavor, use refined coconut oil.

- If the weather is cool you will need to bring the water up to boiling to melt the coconut oil.
- When shopping for Massaman curry paste, look carefully at the carbs and serving size, many pastes are high in sugar.

Massaman Chicken Curry Nutrition Facts			
	(g)	(kcal)	(kcal %)
Fat	148	1329	89%
Carb	15	61	4%
Protein	24	96	6%
		1486	

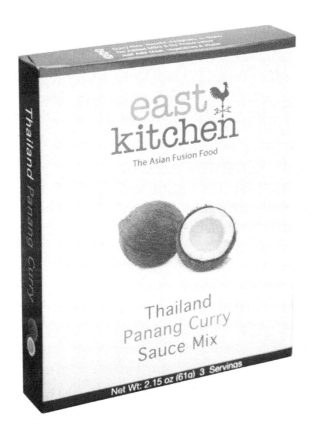

Panang Beef Curry

Prep: Complex
Wilder Ratio: 3.6
Cost/1000kcal: $4.45
kCal/oz: 213

Thick, creamy and spicy, Panang is a classic red curry that packs a punch. Coconut cream smooths out a robust and entertaining mix of Thai flavors including lemongrass, galangal and kaffir lime. Play up your favorite of these of flavors by bringing some extra in dried form.

Ingredients

- 500ml hot water
- 1 packet (12g) Panang Curry paste (East Kitchen)
- 1/2c (24g) freeze dried beef (Valley Food Storage)
- 1/4c (24g) coconut cream powder (Z Natural Foods)
- 1tsp (5g) soy lecithin. Either liquid (Fearn) or powdered (Modernist Pantry)
- 1/4c coconut oil (Nature's Way)
- 1/4c avocado oil (Baja Precious)
- Optional: 2 dried kaffir lime leaves
- Optional: 2 dried galangal leaves
- Optional: 2 dried lemongrass leaves

Process
1. Begin heating the water
2. Mix the beef and Panang curry paste or powder in the water as you heat it, stirring to insure it dissolves.
3. Stir in the extra virgin coconut oil.

Tips:
- Getting pastes and powders to dissolve and blend smoothly on the trail can be difficult. One strategy is to pour all the ingredients into a Nalgene bottle then add an agitator such as a short mini spoon or a few small clean pebbles then shake.
- If you want more texture and can handle the protein, add more beef.
- If you need more calories, keep adding fat until you get to the upper limit of palatability or digestibility. A ¼c of coconut oil is my safe upper limit, I have consumed ½c on several occasions only to have a stomachache and vomit hours later. I think the MCTs are to blame.
- If you need a longer shelf life or don't like the coconut flavor, use refined coconut oil.
- If the weather is cool you will need to bring the water up to boiling to melt the coconut oil.

- When shopping for Panang curry paste, look carefully at the carbs and serving size, many pastes are high in sugar. Same goes for coconut cream powder.

Panang Beef Curry Nutrition Facts			
	(g)	(kcal)	(kcal %)
Fat	141	1266	89%
Carb	20	81	6%
Protein	19	76	5%
		1423	

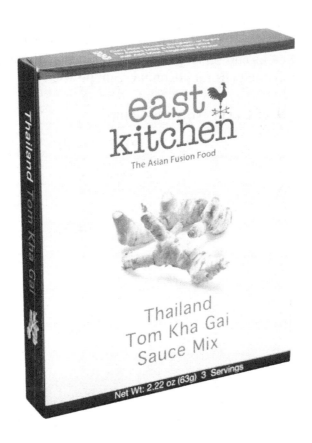

Thai Coconut Chicken Soup (Tom Ka Gai)

Prep: Complex
Wilder Ratio: 2.8
$/1000kcal: $4.72
Kcal/gram: 204

Cool and creamy with fresh notes of lemongrass, this coconut soup is a welcome end to a balmy day. Avocado oil buoys the Wilder ratio but even so, this recipe contains a lot of carbohydrates and is only appropriate for those who produce ketones easily.

Ingredients

- 500ml hot water
- 20g freeze dried chicken (Valley Food Storage)
- 1/3 (25g) packet Tom Ka Gai soup powder (East Kitchen)
- 1/4c (24g) coconut cream powder (Z Natural Foods)
- 1tsp (5g) soy lecithin. Either liquid (Fearn) or powdered (Modernist Pantry)
- 3 tbsp (42g) extra virgin coconut oil
- 3 tbsp (30g) coconut oil powder
- ¼ cup (56g) avocado oil (Baja Precious)
- Optional: Dried Thai birds eye chilis to taste.
- Optional: 2 dried kaffir lime leaves
- Optional: 2 dried galangal leaves
- Optional: 2 dried lemongrass leaves

Process
1. Begin heating water.
2. Add just boiled water to all dry ingredients and stir or shake until no clumps remain.
3. Let sit for 10min until meat has rehydrated.
4. Stir in coconut and avocado oil

Tips:
- Getting pastes and powders to dissolve and blend smoothly on the trail can be difficult. One strategy is to pour all the ingredients into a Nalgene bottle then add an agitator such as a short mini spoon or a few small clean pebbles then shake.
- You can speed up rehydration time for the meat and mushrooms by adding them to the water on the stove, so they hydrate while the water is heating.
- If the Tom Ka Gai powder is already too spicy for you, increase the water or decrease the powder.
- If you need more calories, keep adding fat until you get to the upper limit of palatability or digestibility. A ¼c of coconut oil is my safe upper limit, I have consumed

½ on several occasions only to have a stomachache and vomit hours later.

- If you need a longer shelf life or don't like the coconut flavor, use refined coconut oil.
- If the weather is cool you will need to bring the water up to boiling to melt the coconut oil.
- When shopping for Tom Ka Gai powder, look carefully at the carbs and serving size, many are high in sugar.

Thai Coconut Chicken Soup (Tom Ka Gai) Nutrition Facts			
	(g)	(kcal)	(kcal %)
Fat	147	1320	86%
Carb	25	101	7%
Protein	27	108	7%
		1529	

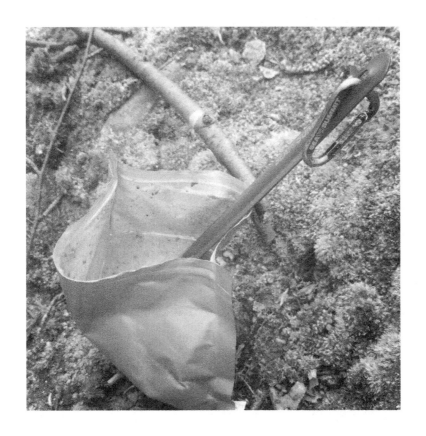

Creamy Tomato Soup v g

Prep: Moderate
Wilder Ratio: 4.2
Cost/$1000kcal: $3.26
Kcal/oz: 194

This tomato soup has a velvety mouth feel and soothing creamy flavor. It's a solid ketogenic meal at a good price.

Ingredients
- 350ml hot water
- 2tbsp (24g) tomato powder (Frontier) or tomato paste from tube (Cento)

- 1tbsp (2g) Italian dry spice blend (or 1tsp dried basil, 1tsp dried parsley and 1tsp dried oregano)
- 4tbsp (48g) heavy cream powder (Anthony's)
- 1tsp (5g) soy lecithin. Either liquid (Fearn) or powdered (Modernist Pantry)
- 4tbsp (57g) olive oil (Trader Joe's)
- 30g grated parmesan cheese (Kraft)

Process
1. Begin heating water.
2. Pour hot water into all dry ingredients and lecithin and stir or shake in a heat resistant bottle such as a Nalgene until dissolved.
3. Add olive oil and shake to mix.

Tips:
- When mixing this from separate ingredients the sequence is very important. Get the dry ingredients well mixed before adding the oil. If you go out of order and develop a surface film of oil, it will be difficult to incorporate.
- I have packed all the ingredients, including the lecithin and olive oil in a single heat-sealed Mylar bag and had a wonderful smooth texture just by adding hot water. I think this is due to the lecithin having time to bind with the oil in the bag.
- The quality of your ingredients will make or break this meal. High quality tomato powder is especially important. Even better is a tube of high quality tomato paste.

Creamy Tomato Soup Nutrition Facts			
	(g)	(kcal)	(kcal %)
Fat	92	828	90%
Carb	18	72	8%
Protein	4	16	2%
		916	

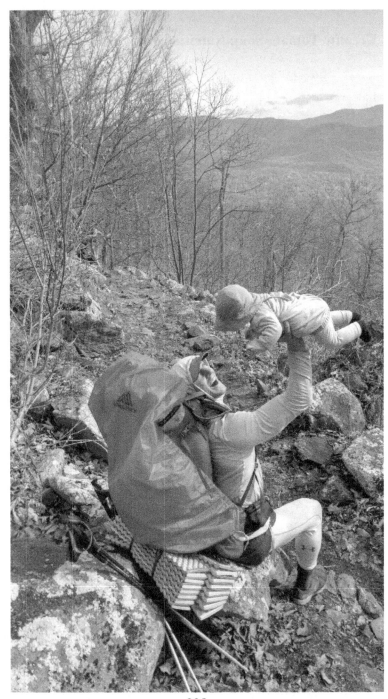

Pepperoni Pizza Soup

Prep: Moderate
Wilder Ratio: 3.2
Cost/1,000kcal: $3.50
Kcal/oz: 177

Hearty slices of tomato and salami in a soup of strong Italian herbs and olive oil. If only there was a flatbread that was low enough in carbs you could boil it down to a sauce and make a pizza.

Ingredients
- 1.5 cups (350ml) of hot water
- 2tbsp (24g) tomato powder (Frontier) or tomato paste from tube (Cento)
- 1tbsp (2g) Italian dry spice blend (or 1tsp dried basil, 1tsp dried parsley and 1tsp dried oregano)
- 1/4c (2g) freeze dried tomatoes (Valley Food Storage)
- 1/2c (114g) olive oil (Trader Joe's)
- 1tsp (5g) soy lecithin. Either liquid (Fearn) or powdered (Modernist Pantry)
- 84g (3oz) sliced pepperoni
- 1/4c (30g) grated parmesan or pecorino Romano (Kraft)

Process
1. Optional: Sauté the pepperoni in two tablespoons of olive oil then remove from pot.
2. Heat water to near boiling.
3. Place all dry ingredients and lecithin in a heat tolerant bottle such as a Nalgene.
4. Pour hot water into bottle, shake and let sit before opening to release pressure.
5. Add olive oil slowly, shaking to incorporate
6. Slowly sprinkle in the cheese, stirring constantly.

Tips:
- When mixing this from separate ingredients the sequence is very important. Get the dry ingredients well mixed before adding the oil. If you go out of order and develop a surface film of oil, it will be difficult to incorporate.
- I have packed all the ingredients, including the lecithin and olive oil in a single heat-sealed Mylar bag and had a wonderful smooth texture just by adding hot water. I think this is due to the lecithin having time to bind with the oil in the bag.
- The quality of your ingredients will make or break this meal. High quality tomato powder is especially important. Even better is a tube of high quality tomato paste.

Pepperoni Pizza Soup Nutrition Facts			
	(g)	(kcal)	(kcal %)
Fat	145	1305	88%
Carb	22	88	6%
Protein	23	92	6%
		1485	

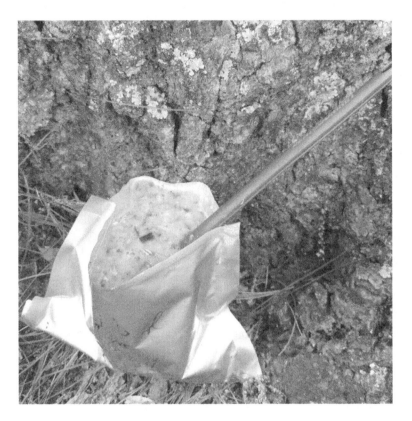

Pork and Cabbage Soup g

Prep: Complex
Wilder Ratio: 2.9
Cost/1,000kcal: $3.58
Kcal/oz: 178

Sweet fennel, chewy cabbage, tangy vinegar, and the rich complex flavor of pastured Mangalitsa lard come together to make this one of my favorite trail dinners.

Ingredients
- 1.5 cups (350ml) hot water
- 1tbsp (7g) onion powder
- 1tbsp (6g) fennel seeds
- 2tbsp apple cider vinegar powder (or 2 vinegar packets)

- 1tbsp mustard powder (or 2 mustard packets)
- 1/2tsp garlic powder
- 1/2tsp black pepper
- 1/4tsp salt
- 1/3c (25g) dehydrated cabbage
- 1/4c (20g) freeze dried sausage crumbles
- 1tsp soy lecithin. Either liquid (Fearn) or powdered (Modernist Pantry)
- 1/2c (102g) lard (pastured Mangalitsa)
- 1oz (28g) grated Pecorino Romano cheese (Trader Joe's)

Process
1. Begin heating the water.
2. Pour all ingredients except lard into Nalgene bottle or bowl.
3. Pour in hot water, shake or stir and wait 5min for meat and cabbage to rehydrate.
4. Add lard and shake or stir to mix.

Tips:
- If mixing ingredients at camp, order is important. Get the dry ingredients well mixed before adding the lard. If you go out of order and develop a surface film of oil, it will be difficult to incorporate.
- I have mixed all ingredients together in the same Mylar bag ahead of time and had no trouble with rehydration or emulsification perhaps because the lecithin and lard have had a lot of time to interact.
- The Mangalitsa breed (also known as the Hungarian Wooly Pig) is prized for it's rich nutty lard and high Omega 3 content when fed a diet of wild plants, nuts and tubers. Use this lard and it will make all the difference. Because of the high PUFA content, oxidation is a concern if stored in a warm environment

for two long. Most of the bags I picked up at mail drops over 1 month old were rancid.

- The relatively low Wilder ratio of this recipe is the result of the high carb content of the cabbage according to its food label. Given the very low carbohydrate content of fresh cabbage, and the high fiber content, this recipe is probably more ketogenic than its Wilder ratio suggests.

Pork and Cabbage Soup Nutrition Facts			
	(g)	(kcal)	(kcal %)
Fat	131	1183	87%
Carb	29	115	8%
Protein	17	68	5%
		1366	

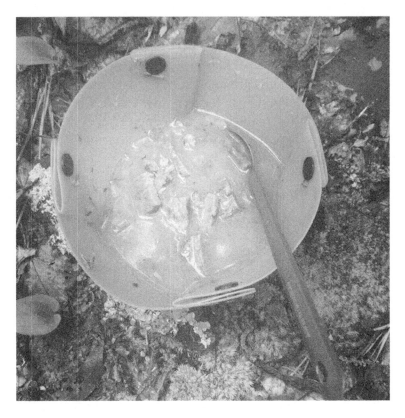

Cheddar Bacon Bisque

Prep: Complex
Wilder Ratio: 2.9
Cost/1,000kcal: $5.61
Kcal/oz: 154

Cheddar and bacon, an all-American combination that will pay back the caloric debt of a day of hard hiking.

- 2 cups (500ml) hot water
- 2tsp chicken bullion
- ½ tsp dried thyme
- ½ tsp garlic powder (consider reducing)
- ½ tsp onion powder

- 10g dehydrated celery
- ¼ tsp cumin
- ¼ tsp pepper
- ¼ tsp cayenne pepper or chili powder for those preferring less spice
- 1tsp (5g) soy lecithin. Either liquid (Fearn) or powdered (Modernist Pantry)
- 2 tbsp (15g) heavy cream powder (Anthony's)
- 4 tbsp (56g) unsalted grass-fed butter (Kerrygold)
- ¼ cup (51g) lard or bacon grease
- 4 oz (112g) cheddar cheese chopped or shredded (Tillamook)
- 2.5 oz (1 small bag, 70g) Bacon bites (Epic)

Process
1. Heat water to boiling
2. Pour water and all ingredients into a bowl and stir until cheese has melted.

Tips:
- You must get the water very hot to melt everything.
- If you aren't too much of a food snob to use bacon bits and cheddar cheese powder it would be cheaper and provide a smoother texture.

Cheddar Bacon Bisque Nutrition Facts			
	(g)	(kcal)	(kcal %)
Fat	169	1520	87%
Carb	7	27	2%
Protein	51	203	12%
		1750	

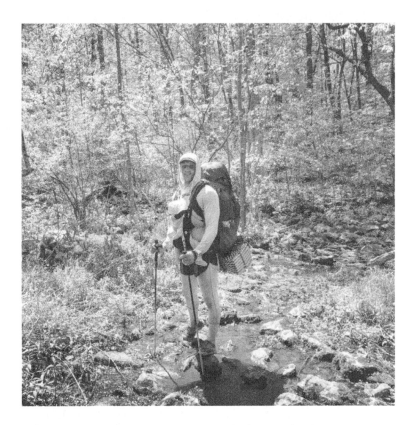

Italian Sausage and Spinach Soup

Prep: Moderate
Wilder Ratio: 3.0
Cost/1,000kcal: $3.95
Kcal/gram: 195

This soup keeps the spice at bay and lets the olive oil and spinach out to play. A substantial dose of spinach packs loads of vitamins. With a pleasant taste and solid stats, keep it in the lineup and you won't be disappointed.

Ingredients
- 2 cups (500ml) hot water
- 1 tbsp (8g) grated parmesan cheese (Kraft)

246

- 1 tsp (1g) Italian seasoning
- 1 tsp basil
- 2 tbsp (24g) sundried tomato powder
- ¼ cup (12g) beef crumbles dehydrated (Valley Food Storage)
- ¼ cup (10g) spinach dehydrated (Harmony House)
- 1tsp (5) soy lecithin. Either liquid (Fearn) or powdered (Modernist Pantry)
- ¼ cup (114g) olive oil (Trader Joe's)

Process
1. Begin heating water.
2. Add hot water to all ingredients except oil in a heat resistant bowl or bottle and stir or shake.
3. Wait 10min for meat to rehydrate.
4. Add olive oil and shake or stir again.

Tips:
- If the olive oil is too strong, use half avocado and half olive oil.

Italian Sausage and Spinach Soup Nutrition Facts			
	(g)	(kcal)	(kcal %)
Fat	115	1032	87%
Carb	22	88	7%
Protein	16	63	5%
		1183	

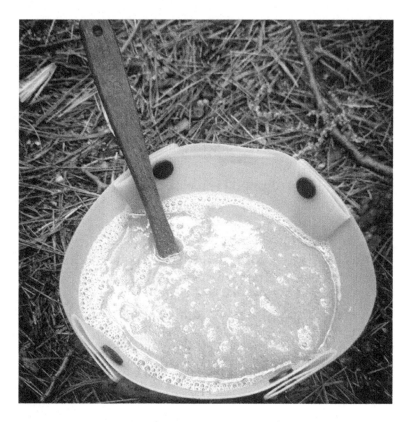

Split Pea Soup

Prep: Moderate
Wilder Ratio: 2.1
Cost/1,000kcal: $2.07
Kcal/gram: 188

Thick, creamy, warm and comforting. Split peas and lard with the zest of olive oil. This recipe is a template for pairing the lower carb versions of backpacking friendly dehydrated soup mixes with a complementary fat source. Even with the addition of 1/2c of fat, the Wilder ratio of this recipe is still on the low end and this recipe is only appropriate for those who can handle a decent amount of carbs without impairing fat burning.

Ingredients

- 2 cups (500ml) hot water
- ½ cup dehydrated split pea soup mix (Berkeley Bowl)
- 1tsp (5g) soy lecithin. Either liquid (Fearn) or powdered (Modernist Pantry)
- ¼ cup (51g) pastured lard (Mangalitsa)
- ¼ cup (114g) olive oil (Trader Joe's)

Process

1. Begin heating water.
2. Add hot water to all ingredients except olive oil and lard in a heat resistant bowl or bottle and stir or shake.
3. Add olive oil and lard and shake or stir again.

Tips:

- If the olive oil is too strong, use half avocado and half olive oil.
- This recipe can be simplified by using just lard.

Split Pea Soup Nutrition Facts			
	(g)	(kcal)	(kcal %)
Fat	109	983	83%
Carb	38	152	13%
Protein	14	56	5%
		1191	

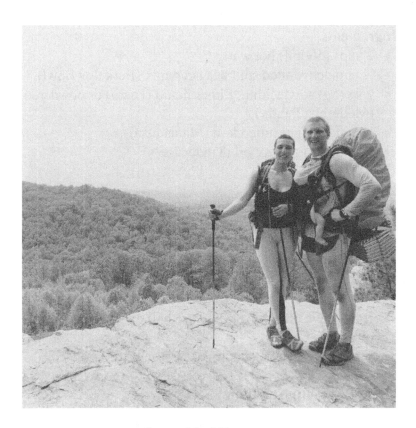

Scrambled Eggs p v g

Prep: Moderate
Wilder Ratio: 2.8
Cost/1,000kcal: $4.04
Kcal/oz: 186

Scrambled eggs cooked in butter makes a hearty backcountry breakfast that will stick to your ribs… and to the pot.

Ingredients
- 1/4c (125ml) water
- 6tbsp (39g) dry eggs powder (Gluten Free You and Me)
- 4tbsp (56g) grass fed salted butter (Kerrygold)

- Salt and pepper to taste

Process
1. Mix egg and water in a cup
2. Melt butter in pan over low heat
3. Once butter is melted, pour in eggs and stir immediately with a spatula to prevent sticking.
4. Cook slowly over low heat with constant stirring to incorporate butter and eggs.

Tips
- I don't recommend attempting this unless you have a stove capable of adjustable low heat and a non-stick pan. Cleaning egg off a pan is not a chore I look forward to even where there is a sink present.

Scrambled Eggs Nutrition Facts			
	(g)	(kcal)	(kcal %)
Fat	59	531	86%
Carb	3	12	2%
Protein	18	72	12%
		615	

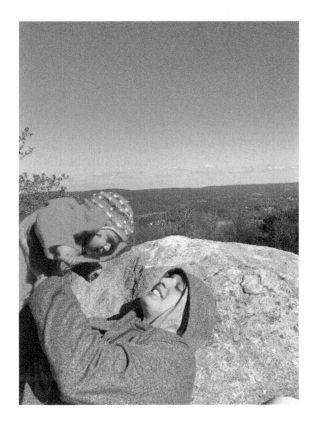

Scrambled Eggs and Sausage

Prep: Complex
Wilder Ratio: 2.5
Cost/1,000kcal: $5.92
Kcal/oz: 189

Repair and rebuild with a protein- packed mess of eggs and sausage. Add mushrooms and peppers to make it a party.

Ingredients
- ½ (250ml) cup hot water
- 4tbsp (56g) grass fed salted butter (Kerrygold)
- 6tbsp (39g) dry eggs powder (Gluten Free You and Me)
  1/2 cup (40g) freeze dried sausage (Valley Food Storage)

- ¼ tsp salt
- 1/2tsp pepper
- 10g oyster mushrooms dried (optional)
- 10g freeze dried bell peppers (optional)

Process
1. Heat ½ cup of water to near boiling.
2. Mix dry eggs and sausage in a small cup and slowly pour in hot water while stirring.
3. Stir and wait 10min to rehydrate.
4. Mix in butter.

Tips
- The challenge with this recipe is getting the egg powder to dissolve fully without clumps.
- If adding mushrooms and peppers, increase the water by 2tbsp.
- This recipe is too high in protein for most to stay in ketosis. Add more butter on top if you want to be sure of staying in ketosis.

Eggs and Sausage Nutrition Facts			
	(g)	(kcal)	(kcal %)
Fat	84	756	85%
Carb	4	16	2%
Protein	30	120	13%
		911	

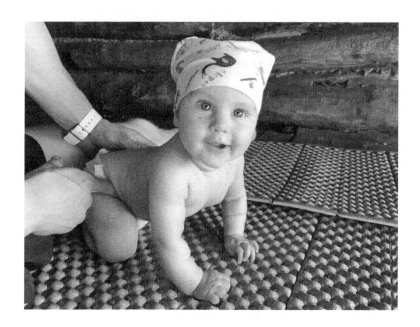

Broccoli and Butter p v g

Prep: Complex
Wilder Ratio: 3.7
Cost/1,000kcal: $5.10
Kcal/oz: 176

This delicious combination is a trailside recreation of the ketogenic staple buttered veggies. The same format can be applied to cauliflower, artichokes, asparagus and any other low-carb vegetable that you can find in freeze dried form.

Ingredients
- ½ cup (250ml) hot water
- 1 oz (28g) freed dried broccoli (Mother Earth Products)
- 4tbsp (56g) grass fed salted butter (Kerrygold)
- Salt and pepper to taste

Process
1. Heat ½ cup of water to near boiling.

2. Pour hot water on broccoli and wait several minutes to rehydrate.
3. Drink excess water (no reason to waste water and vitamins)
4. Add butter, salt and pepper to taste.

Tips
- Tame your expectations, freeze dried vegetables just aren't the same as fresh or frozen vegetables.

Broccoli and Butter Nutrition Facts			
	(g)	(kcal)	(kcal %)
Fat	45	401	89%
Carb	8	30	7%
Protein	5	18	4%
		449	

21. Trailmade Recipes- Sweet

This collection of delicious warm and sweet beverages will boost your spirits no matter how dreary the weather. With only trace amounts of carbs and protein, they are highly ketogenic. I spent countless hours on these recipes trying different ingredients and ratios to produce the best flavor and mouth feel while still delivering enough fat to power a morning of hiking. The first few versions of hot chocolate I made were undrinkable and had to be thrown out. But my recipes improved over the course of the ten weeks between when our daughter was born and when we set out on the Appalachian trail. I made a different version of hot chocolate nearly every morning for my wife. Through her critique and constant improvement, I arrived at recipes that were so good she packed hot chocolate for nearly half of her morning meals on the Appalachian Trail. Our daughter who has been nursing this whole time must be made of chocolate milk.

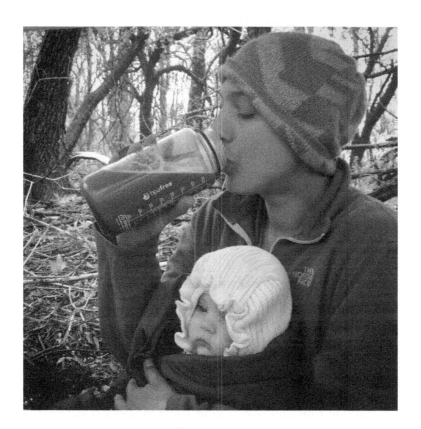

Hazelnut Hot Chocolate p v g vegan

Prep: Complex
Wilder Ratio: 11
Cost/1,000kcal: $2.17
Kcal/oz: 220

A cold wind and driving rain are no match for a thermos of hot chocolate fuel. A robust dark chocolate flavor is followed by sweet and nutty hazelnut.

Ingredients

- 3 cups (700ml) hot water
- ½ tsp liquid vanilla extract or vanilla powder or 2cm dried vanilla bean

- 3 tbsp (15g) chocolate powder (Wild brand)
- 1tsp stevia (Trader Joe's)
- 1tsp (5g) soy lecithin. Either liquid (Fearn) or powdered (Modernist Pantry)
- ½ cup (112g) hazelnut oil (La Tourangelle)
- Optional Mexican Style: ¼ tsp chili powder and ¼ tsp cinnamon
- Optional Winter Spice: ¼ tsp cinnamon, ¼ teaspoon cloves, ¼ tsp allspice

Process

Method 1: Pack Chocolate and Oil Together in a Mylar Bag
1. Pack all ingredients except water in a heat-tolerant Mylar bag and seal.
2. Pour contents of bag into a heat tolerant thermos or water bottle.
3. Heat water.
4. When water has reached desired temperature, pour half into thermos and shake. Pour the remaining water into the bag and stir to release the remaining chocolate, then pour this into the Nalgene and shake.
5. Let sit for 1 min to allow pressure to decrease before opening.

Method 2: Pack Chocolate and Oil Separately
1. Make your own "hot chocolate powder" by mixing all the dry ingredients for several servings in a large bag. Use vanilla powder or vanilla bean and powdered soy lecithin.
2. Pack oil separately in a leakproof bottle.
3. Pour desired amount of chocolate powder into a heat tolerant thermos or water bottle.
4. Heat water.

5. When water has reached desired temperature, pour into thermos and shake. Once mixed, pour in desired amount of oil and shake gain.
6. Let sit for 1 min to allow pressure to decrease before opening.

Tips
- If you are starting with clean water, you can save water and fuel and reduce the risk of burning yourself by heating the water only up to the desired temperature.
- The key to flavor is starting with excellent cocoa powder, I tried many brands and only Wild Foods resulted in a hot chocolate I liked.
- Among the nut oils I have found that hazelnut as the strongest and most pleasant flavor but experiment with different nut oils to find the one you like best.
- If you don't need as many calories, you can cut the amount of oil in half and the result will still be highly ketogenic.

Hazelnut Hot Chocolate Nutrition Facts			
	(g)	(kcal)	(kcal %)
Fat	114	1022	96%
Carb	8	30	3%
Protein	3	12	1%
		1064	

259

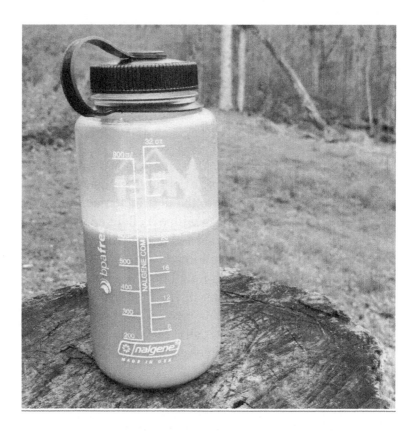

Cheater's Hot Chocolate p v g vegan

Prep: Complex
Wilder Ratio: 2.1
Cost/1,000kcal: $7.15
Kcal/oz: 166

Loaded with medium chain triglycerides which are directly converted to ketones, this hot chocolate is highly ketogenic despite its low Wilder ratio, hence the name Cheater's. In addition to providing immediate energy, this chocolate has a wonderfully creamy mouth feel and if you work hard enough at it you can whip up a frothy head. If it sounds too good to be true, look at the price.

Ingredients
- 3 cups (700ml) hot water
- ½ tsp vanilla powder or 2cm dried vanilla bean
- 3 tbsp (15g) chocolate powder (Wild brand)
- 3 scoops (27g) of MCT oil powder (Quest)
- 3 scoops (30g) of coconut oil powder (Quest)
- 1tsp stevia (Trader Joe's)
- 1tsp soy lecithin powdered (Modernist Pantry)

Process
1. Make your own "hot chocolate powder" by mixing all the dry ingredients for several servings in a large bag. Pack oil separately in a leakproof bottle.
2. Scoop desired amount of chocolate powder into a heat tolerant thermos or water bottle.
3. Heat water.
4. When water has reached desired temperature, pour into thermos and shake.
5. Let sit for 1 min to allow pressure to decrease before opening.

Tips
- Getting all these powders to dissolve and blend smoothly on the trail can be difficult and may leave you crying out for an immersion blender. One strategy is to add an agitator such as a short mini spoon or a few small clean pebbles to the bottle then shake.
- If you are starting with clean water, you can save water and fuel and reduce the risk of burning yourself by heating the water only up to the desired temperature.
- The key to flavor is starting with excellent cocoa powder, I tried many brands and only Wild Foods resulted in a hot chocolate I liked.

Cheater's Hot Chocolate Nutrition Facts			
	(g)	(kcal)	(kcal %)
Fat	47	419	82%
Carb	17	66	13%
Protein	6	24	5%
		509	

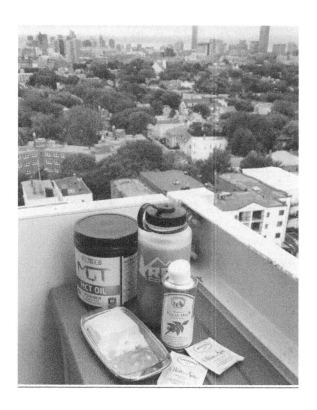

Winter Spice Tea p v g

Prep: Complex
Wilder Ratio: zero carbs and protein
Cost/1,000kcal: $6.96
Kcal/oz: 195

Warmth and comfort in a bottle. Delight in the soft aroma
of chamomile, cinnamon and cloves and the soothing warm
and nutty flavors of butter and pecan oil.

Ingredients
- 3 cups (700ml) hot water
- 2 bags of winter spice tea (Twinning's)
- 1.5 tsp stevia (Trader Joe's)
- 4 tbsp (56g) grass-fed unsalted butter (Kerrygold)

263

- 4 tbsp (56g) pecan oil (La Tourangelle)
- Optional: 1tsp (5g) soy lecithin. Either liquid (Fearn) or powdered (Modernist Pantry)

Process
1. Begin heating water.
2. When water nears boiling, turn off heat and place tea bags in water. Steep for 6min, longer for stronger flavor.
3. When tea is done steeping, remove bags and pour tea into Nalgene with stevia, butter, pecan oil and lecithin. Seal and shake to mix.
4. Wait for pressure to settle before opening.

Tips
- If you forego the lecithin, you will need to shake periodically before drinking
- You can simplify this recipe by removing the butter and using only pecan oil. Other nut oils can be substituted as well.
- If you are starting with clean water, you can save water and fuel and reduce the risk of burning yourself by heating the water only up to the desired temperature.

Winter Spice Tea Nutrition Facts			
	(g)	(kcal)	(kcal %)
Fat	100	900	100%
Carb			0%
Protein			0%
		864	

264

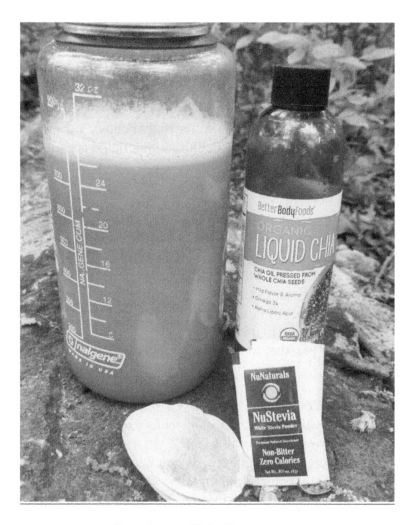

Raspberry Chia Tea p v g vegan

Prep: Complex
Wilder Ratio: zero carbs and protein
Cost/1,000kcal: $6.83
Kcal/oz: 224

Sweet raspberry and nutty chia seed combine to start your morning off with a bottle full of healthy fats and antioxidants.

Ingredients
- 3 cups (700ml) hot water
- 3bags of raspberry goji berry green tea (Bigelow)
- 1.5 tsp stevia (Trader Joe's)
- 1/2c (96g) chia seed oil (Better Body Foods)
- Optional: 1tsp (5g) soy lecithin. Either liquid (Fearn) or powdered (Modernist Pantry)

Process
1. Begin heating water.
2. When water nears boiling, turn off heat and place tea bags in water. Steep for 6min, longer for stronger flavor.
3. When tea is done steeping, remove bags and pour tea into Nalgene with stevia, chia seed oil and lecithin.
4. Seal and shake to mix.
5. Wait for pressure to settle before opening.

Tips
- Chia oil comes in convenient 8oz bottles that are relatively light, are shelf stable before opening and will make two servings of this tea.
- If you forego the lecithin, you will need to shake periodically before drinking
- If you are starting with clean water, you can save water and fuel and reduce the risk of burning yourself by heating the water only up to the desired temperature.

Raspberry Chia Tea Nutrition Facts			
	(g)	(kcal)	(kcal %)
Fat	96	864	100%
Carb			0%
Protein			0%
		864	

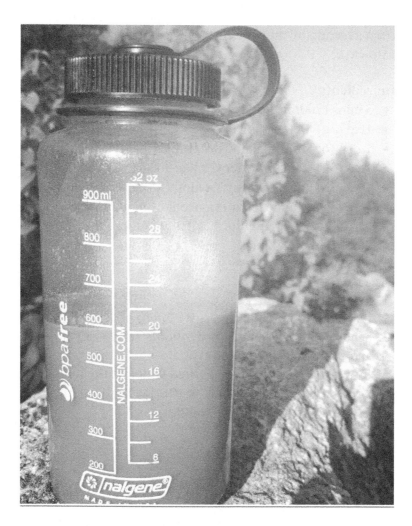

Hippie Green Drink p v g vegan

Prep: Complex
Wilder Ratio: 30.4
Cost/1,000kcal: $3.37
Kcal/oz: 220

A ketogenic breakfast to make any hippie green with envy.
Green tea meets smoothie in this energizing blend of

Matcha tea, antioxidant rich moringa powder, healthy fats from avocado oil and sweetness from apple and stevia leaf extract.

Ingredients
- 3 cups (700ml) hot water
- 1tsp (3g) matcha powder (Zen Spirit)
- 1tbsp (6g) moringa powder (Maju)
- 1tsp (3g) stevia powder (Trader Joe's)
- 1tsp (5g) powdered soy lecithin (Modernist Pantry)
- 1/2c (112g) avocado oil (make it even greener by partially exchanging for hemp seed oil)
- 2 drops apple extract

Process
1. Begin heating water.
2. Place dry ingredients and soy lecithin in the bottom of a heat tolerant thermos or water bottle such as a Nalgene and shake lightly to mix.
3. When water has reached desired temperature, pour hot water into bottle and shake or stir. Let sit 1min, then open slowly to release pressure.
4. Add oil and shake or stir again.

Tips
- If you are starting with clean water, you can save water and fuel and reduce the risk of burning yourself by heating the water only up to the desired temperature.
- I have packed all the dry ingredients and oil in a Mylar bag and heat sealed it, then added hot water on the trail. This resulted in a very smooth texture, perhaps because the soy lecithin bound to the oil while in the bag.

Hippie Green Drink Nutrition Facts			
	(g)	(kcal)	(kcal %)
Fat	116	1041	99%
Carb	0	1	0%
Protein	4	14	1%
		1056	

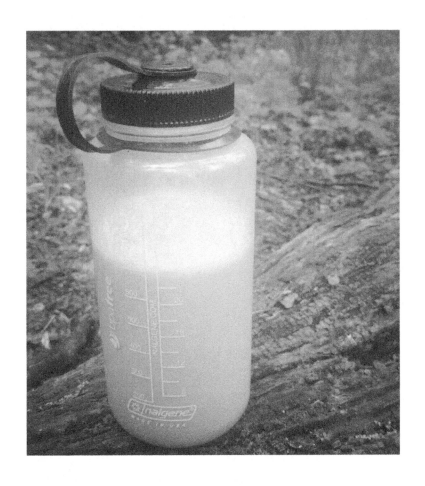

Creamy Chai p v g

Prep: Moderate
Wilder Ratio: Zero carbs and protein
Cost/1,000kcal: $5.46
Kcal/oz: 201

A blend of aromatic spices balance with a robust black tea on a complex background of cream and butter with sweet butterscotch notes of ghee.

Ingredients

- 3 cups (700ml) hot water
- 2 bags of chai tea (Tazo)
- 4 tbsp (48g) heavy cream powder (Anthony's)
- ½ tsp stevia (Trader Joe's)
- 2 tbsp (28g) unsalted grass-fed butter (Kerrygold)
- 2 tbsp (30g) unsalted grass-fed ghee (Banyan Botanicals)

Process

1. Heat water to near boiling
2. Place tea bags in thermos or heat tolerant water bottle such as a Nalgene.
3. Steep tea for 6min then remove tea bags.
4. Add cream powder, stevia butter and ghee then shake vigorously.
5. Wait 1 minute then loosen seal carefully to release pressure.

Tips

- If you like ghee, you can simplify the recipe by excluding the butter and using only ghee and cream.
- If you don't need as many calories, you can simplify the recipe by excluding the butter and ghee and only using the heavy cream powder.
- MCT oil powder is a good addition or substitute for the heavy cream powder to guarantee ketone production.
- If you are starting with clean water, you can save fuel and time by just heating the water up just shy of boiling.

Creamy Chai Nutrition Facts			
	(g)	(kcal)	(kcal %)
Fat	88	792	100%
Carb	0	0	0%
Protein	0	0	0%
		792	

VI. TABLES AND FIGURES

Backpacking Foods Sorted by Calories per Ounce.

In this table you can see all the recipes in this book as well as twenty-three popular backpacking foods sorted by their weight efficiency as measured by the number of calories they contain per ounce. The results are clear, the recipes in this book are dramatically more efficient than standard backpacking foods. The recipes in this book that score the lowest are those that contain a lot of meat, but even these beat the standard high carb backpacking meals. The only exception is peanut butter, due to it high fat content, it scores much better than other standard backpacking foods.

You may be surprised to find that freeze-dried backpacking meals score as low on weight efficiency as other backpacking standards. These meals feel so light, they seem like they would be synonymous with ultra-light backpacking. Indeed, they are light, but in addition to lacking water, they don't contain that many calories. This should come as no surprise as the problem of fat oxidation in long term food storage means that most of these meals are relatively low in fat.

Beef jerky is another food that is a perennial backpacking favorite, but it fails miserably in providing calories. Its only advantage is providing protein, variety and good shelf life.

Backpacking Foods Sorted by Calories per Ounce

Name	kCal/oz	$/1000kcal	Wilder
Smoky Apple Walnut Whip	232	$1.71	8.1
Thai Beef Bone Broth- LonoLife	232	$5.41	6.5
Turmeric Ginger Tea	230	$2.43	359.0
Raspberry Chia Tea	224	$6.83	#DIV/0!
Hippie Green Drink	222	$3.37	30.4
Walnut Maple Cream	221	$2.49	8.4
Triple Mushroom Soup	221	$3.17	10.5
Hazelnut Hot Chocolate	220	$2.17	10.8
Bacon, Bison, and Blueberry Pemmican	218	$7.80	9.4
Spicy Sesame Mushroom Soup	217	$5.93	2.8
Thai Cashew Butter- Traer Joe's Cashew Butter	217	$2.07	5.3
Matsutake Soup	216	$8.19	8.4
Bean-less Hummus	216	$2.03	5.9
Cashews in Seasoned Ghee	214	$2.04	3.9
Thai Cashew Butter- Sunbelt Raw Cashews	214	$1.98	4.3
Walnut Hot Chocolate	214	$2.56	8.1
Panang Beef Curry	213	$4.45	3.6
Green and Black's Almond Fudge	213	$4.98	4.1
Massaman Chicken Curry	213	$3.72	3.8
Pome Mac Jetpack	212	$4.30	4.9
Seasoned Buffalo Ghee and Cashew Butter	212	$2.21	4.1

Thai Cashew Butter- Trader Joe's Chili Lime Cashews	212	$2.05	4.2
Machacado Lardican	211	$4.12	4.3
Coconut Chocolate Trailmix with Green & Black's 85%	210	$5.46	3.0
Thai Hot and Sour Soup (Tom Yum)	207	$3.16	4.2
Black Tea with Buffalo Butter	206	$1.88	#DIV/0!
Chocolate Hazelnut Cream	206	$3.30	5.0
Thai Coconut Chicken Soup (Tom Ka Gai)	204	$4.72	2.8
Dark Pine Trail Mix Green & Blacks 85%	202	$5.27	3.0
Creamy Chai	201	$5.46	#DIV/0!
Peanut Cream	201	$2.01	3.2
Lindt's Peanut Fudge	200	$4.54	3.6
Peanut Cream with Cacao Nibs	199	$3.31	2.9
Dark Pine Trail Mix with Montezuma's Absolute Black	198	$4.72	4.9
Montezuma's Absolute Black Fudge	196	$3.98	4.8
Salmon Skin Chips and Mayo	196	$5.83	8.9
Winter Spice Tea	195	$6.96	#DIV/0!
Italian Spinach and Sausage Soup	195	$3.95	3.0
Bacon's Heir Pork Clouds and Mayo	195	$3.86	6.1
Galactic Hog Skins and Mayo	195	$5.45	8.0
4505 Chicharrones and Mayo	195	$6.41	6.1
Creamy Tomato Soup	194	$3.26	4.2
Pork Crackling's and Mayo	194	$6.16	6.6
Parmesan Pesto	191	$3.43	3.8

Seaweed Maw Soup	191	$6.81	3.2
Scrambled Eggs and Sausage	189	$5.92	2.5
Moon Cheese and Butter	188	$5.60	4.1
Split Pea Soup	188	$2.07	2.1
Coconut Chocolate Trailmix with Choczero 92%	187	$6.11	3.1
Buttered Broth- Protein Essentials	186	$4.10	6.1
Scrambled Eggs	186	$4.04	2.8
Bacon, Bison, and Cherry Pemmican	186	$6.29	4.0
Buttered Broth- LonoLife	186	$4.42	6.8
Buttered Broth- Orrington	185	$2.42	14.8
BBQ Protein Chips and Mayo	185	$4.17	4.2
Peanut Butter	183	$1.67	2.9
Almond Butter	183	$2.55	3.0
Cashew Butter Butter	183	$2.55	3.2
Pork and Cabbage Soup	178	$3.58	2.9
Salami, Lard, and Mustard	178	$2.85	4.9
Pepperoni Pizza Soup	177	$3.50	3.2
Machacado and Beef Tallow Pemmican	176	$10.58	1.4
Broccoli and Butter	176	$5.10	3.7
Toscano, Lard, and Salmon	169	$4.23	3.7
Peanut Butter	166	$0.78	1.2
Cheater's Hot Chocolate	166	$7.15	2.1
Chorizo, Roncal, and Goat's Milk Butter	164	$5.70	4.3
Cheddar Bacon Soup	154	$5.61	2.9

Pepperoni Swiss Rolls	152	$6.72	3.2
Cheddar, Butter, and Cherry	152	$2.75	3.1
Trail Mix- Peanuts, Raisins, M & Ms, Almonds and Cashews	149	$1.30	0.5
Ritz Cracker Sandwiches	144	$1.86	0.4
Smoked Gouda, Butter and Apple	144	$3.38	2.4
Asiago, Butter, and Olive	140	$4.68	4.7
Oreo Double Stuf	135	$1.28	0.3
Goldfish	131	$1.60	0.2
Nori Fish Wraps	130	$3.54	5.4
Beef Stroganoff with Noodles	128	$8.36	0.3
Instant Ramen Noodles	127	$2.00	0.2
Oats and Honey Granola Bars	127	$2.32	0.2
Swiss Rolls (2 count)	124	$0.62	0.3
Chili Mac with Beef	119	$8.43	0.1
Skittles	112	$1.87	0.0
3z Glazed Honey Bun	112	$3.19	0.3
Pop-Tart Frosted Strawberry (1 count)	108	$1.63	0.1
Easy Mac	106	$3.23	0.1
Swedish Fish	105	$1.99	0.0
Rice Sides- Chicken Rice and Pasta Blend	102	$1.65	0.0
Plain Bagel- Thomas Brand	102	$1.65	0.0
Snicker's Bar Full Size	102	$1.65	0.3
Instant Oatmeal	100	$2.20	0.1
Fig Newtons	100	$2.29	0.1
Twinkies (2 count)	98	$2.15	0.2

Beef Jerky- Jack Link's	80	$17.13	0.1
Red Beans and Rice-dehydrated	98	$7.60	0.0
*Classic Backpacking Foods Highlighted in Grey			

Backpacking Foods Sorted by Price

Although the ketogenic backpacking foods in this book are much more weight efficient than standard high-carb foods, they are consistently more expensive. This is not an entirely fair comparison, as the ingredients in the recipes in this book have been chosen for their health properties, not their price. Cheaper ketogenic meals could be made primarily by using vegetable oils and still be healthier than the junk most backpackers are eating.

This table reveals a fact well known to thru hikers: freeze dried meals are exorbitantly expensive. Combined with their poor kcal/oz scores, their only benefit is their ease of preparation and semblance of a normal meal. You can see why most thru hikers consider them a luxury food.

Beef jerky also fails miserably in price, providing very few calories for a lot of dollars.

The clear winner in cost is peanut butter. This combined with the fact that it beats all other standard backpacking food in kcal/oz, (but still far behind most ketogenic foods) explain why so many thru hikers live on, and get sick of peanut and other nut butters.

Backpacking Foods Sorted by Cost per 1,000 kcal

Name	kCal/oz	$/1000kcal	Wilder
Swiss Rolls (2 count)	124	$0.62	0.3
Peanut Butter	166	$0.78	1.2
Oreo Double Stuf	135	$1.28	0.3
Trail Mix- Peanuts, Raisins, M & Ms, Almonds and Cashews	149	$1.30	0.5
Goldfish	131	$1.60	0.2
Pop-Tart Frosted Strawberry (1 count)	108	$1.63	0.1
Snicker's Bar Full Size	102	$1.65	0.3
Rice Sides- Chicken Rice and Pasta Blend	102	$1.65	0.0
Plain Bagel- Thomas Brand	102	$1.65	0.0
Peanut Butter Butter	183	$1.67	2.9
Smoky Apple Walnut Whip	232	$1.71	8.1
Ritz Cracker Sandwiches	144	$1.86	0.4
Skittles	112	$1.87	0.0
Black Tea with Buffalo Butter	206	$1.88	#DIV/0!
Thai Cashew Butter- Sunbelt Raw Cashews	214	$1.98	4.3
Swedish Fish	105	$1.99	0.0
Instant Ramen Noodles	127	$2.00	0.2
Peanut Cream	201	$2.01	3.2

Bean-less Hummus	216	$2.03	5.9
Cashews in Seasoned Ghee	214	$2.04	3.9
Thai Cashew Butter- Trader Joe's Chili Lime Cashews	212	$2.05	4.2
Thai Cashew Butter- Traer Joe's Cashew Butter	217	$2.07	5.3
Split Pea Soup	188	$2.07	2.1
Twinkies (2 count)	98	$2.15	0.2
Hazelnut Hot Chocolate	220	$2.17	10.8
Instant Oatmeal	100	$2.20	0.1
Seasoned Buffalo Ghee and Cashew Butter	212	$2.21	4.1
Fig Newtons	100	$2.29	0.1
Oats and Honey Granola Bars	127	$2.32	0.2
Buttered Broth- Orrington	185	$2.42	14.8
Turmeric Ginger Tea	230	$2.43	359.0
Walnut Maple Cream	221	$2.49	8.4
Cashew Butter Butter	183	$2.55	3.2
Almond Butter Butter	183	$2.55	3.0
Walnut Hot Chocolate	214	$2.56	8.1
Cheddar, Butter, and Cherry	152	$2.75	3.1
Salami, Lard, and Mustard	178	$2.85	4.9
Thai Hot and Sour Soup (Tom Yum)	207	$3.16	4.2
Triple Mushroom Soup	221	$3.17	10.5
3z Glazed Honey Bun	112	$3.19	0.3
Easy Mac	106	$3.23	0.1
Creamy Tomato Soup	194	$3.26	4.2

Chocolate Hazelnut Cream	206	$3.30	5.0
Peanut Cream with Cacao Nibs	199	$3.31	2.9
Hippie Green Drink	222	$3.37	30.4
Smoked Gouda, Butter and Apple	144	$3.38	2.4
Parmesan Pesto	191	$3.43	3.8
Pepperoni Pizza Soup	177	$3.50	3.2
Nori Fish Wraps	130	$3.54	5.4
Pork and Cabbage Soup	178	$3.58	2.9
Massaman Chicken Curry	213	$3.72	3.8
Bacon's Heir Pork Clouds and Mayo	195	$3.86	6.1
Italian Spinach and Sausage Soup	195	$3.95	3.0
Montezuma's Absolute Black Fudge	196	$3.98	4.8
Scrambled Eggs	186	$4.04	2.8
Buttered Broth- Protein Essentials	186	$4.10	6.1
Machacado Lardican	211	$4.12	4.3
BBQ Protein Chips and Mayo	185	$4.17	4.2
Toscano, Lard, and Salmon	169	$4.23	3.7
Pome Mac Jetpack	212	$4.30	4.9
Buttered Broth- LonoLife	186	$4.42	6.8
Panang Beef Curry	213	$4.45	3.6
Lindt's Peanut Fudge	200	$4.54	3.6
Asiago, Butter, and Olive	140	$4.68	4.7
Dark Pine Trail Mix with Montezuma's Absolute Black	198	$4.72	4.9
Thai Coconut Chicken Soup (Tom Ka Gai)	204	$4.72	2.8

Green and Black's Almond Fudge	213	$4.98	4.1
Broccoli and Butter	176	$5.10	3.7
Dark Pine Trail Mix Green & Blacks 85%	202	$5.27	3.0
Thai Beef Bone Broth- LonoLife	232	$5.41	6.5
Galactic Hog Skins and Mayo	195	$5.45	8.0
Creamy Chai	201	$5.46	#DIV/0!
Coconut Chocolate Trailmix with Green & Black's 85%	210	$5.46	3.0
Moon Cheese and Butter	188	$5.60	4.1
Cheddar Bacon Soup	154	$5.61	2.9
Chorizo, Roncal, and Goat's Milk Butter	164	$5.70	4.3
Salmon Skin Chips and Mayo	196	$5.83	8.9
Scrambled Eggs and Sausage	189	$5.92	2.5
Spicy Sesame Mushroom Soup	217	$5.93	2.8
Coconut Chocolate Trailmix with Choczero 92%	187	$6.11	3.1
Pork Crackling's and Mayo	194	$6.16	6.6
Bacon, Bison, and Cherry Pemmican	186	$6.29	4.0
4505 Chicharrones and Mayo	195	$6.41	6.1
Pepperoni Swiss Rolls	152	$6.72	3.2
Seaweed Maw Soup	191	$6.81	3.2
Raspberry Chia Tea	224	$6.83	#DIV/0!
Winter Spice Tea	195	$6.96	#DIV/0!
Cheater's Hot Chocolate	166	$7.15	2.1
Red Beans and Rice	98	$7.60	0.0
Bacon, Bison, and Blueberry Pemmican	218	$7.80	9.4

Matsutake Soup	216	$8.19	8.4
Beef Stroganoff with Noodles	128	$8.36	0.3
Chili Mac with Beef	119	$8.43	0.1
Machacado and Beef Tallow Pemmican	176	$10.58	1.4
Beef Jerky- Jack Link's	80	$17.13	0.1
*Classic Backpacking Foods Highlighted in Grey			

Backpacking Foods Sorted by Wilder Ratio

You will find this table useful when planning your ketogenic diet. The meals with the highest wilder ratio are the hot beverages, some of these contain no carbohydrates or protein and thus the Wilder ratio cannot be calculated. None of the classic backpacking favorites are remotely ketogenic. In the modern food environment, a ketogenic diet is not something you stumble across by accident.

Backpacking Foods Sorted by Wilder Ratio			
Name	kCal/oz	$/1000kcal	Wilder
Black Tea with Buffalo Butter	206	$1.88	#DIV/0!
Creamy Chai	201	$5.46	#DIV/0!
Raspberry Chia Tea	224	$6.83	#DIV/0!
Winter Spice Tea	195	$6.96	#DIV/0!
Turmeric Ginger Tea	230	$2.43	359.0
Hippie Green Drink	222	$3.37	30.4
Buttered Broth- Orrington	185	$2.42	14.8
Hazelnut Hot Chocolate	220	$2.17	10.8
Triple Mushroom Soup	221	$3.17	10.5

Bacon, Bison, and Blueberry Pemmican	218	$7.80	9.4
Salmon Skin Chips and Mayo	196	$5.83	8.9
Matsutake Soup	216	$8.19	8.4
Walnut Maple Cream	221	$2.49	8.4
Walnut Hot Chocolate	214	$2.56	8.1
Smoky Apple Walnut Whip	232	$1.71	8.1
Galactic Hog Skins and Mayo	195	$5.45	8.0
Buttered Broth- LonoLife	186	$4.42	6.8
Pork Crackling's and Mayo	194	$6.16	6.6
Thai Beef Bone Broth- LonoLife	232	$5.41	6.5
Bacon's Heir Pork Clouds and Mayo	195	$3.86	6.1
4505 Chicharrones and Mayo	195	$6.41	6.1
Buttered Broth- Protein Essentials	186	$4.10	6.1
Bean-less Hummus	216	$2.03	5.9
Nori Fish Wraps	130	$3.54	5.4
Thai Cashew Butter- Traer Joe's Cashew Butter	217	$2.07	5.3
Chocolate Hazelnut Cream	206	$3.30	5.0
Salami, Lard, and Mustard	178	$2.85	4.9
Dark Pine Trail Mix with Montezuma's Absolute Black	198	$4.72	4.9
Pome Mac Jetpack	212	$4.30	4.9
Montezuma's Absolute Black Fudge	196	$3.98	4.8
Asiago, Butter, and Olive	140	$4.68	4.7
Thai Cashew Butter- Sunbelt Raw Cashews	214	$1.98	4.3

Chorizo, Roncal, and Goat's Milk Butter	164	$5.70	4.3
Machacado Lardican	211	$4.12	4.3
Thai Hot and Sour Soup (Tom Yum)	207	$3.16	4.2
Thai Cashew Butter- Trader Joe's Chili Lime Cashews	212	$2.05	4.2
Creamy Tomato Soup	194	$3.26	4.2
BBQ Protein Chips and Mayo	185	$4.17	4.2
Green and Black's Almond Fudge	213	$4.98	4.1
Moon Cheese and Butter	188	$5.60	4.1
Seasoned Buffalo Ghee and Cashew Butter	212	$2.21	4.1
Bacon, Bison, and Cherry Pemmican	186	$6.29	4.0
Cashews in Seasoned Ghee	214	$2.04	3.9
Massaman Chicken Curry	213	$3.72	3.8
Parmesan Pesto	191	$3.43	3.8
Broccoli and Butter	176	$5.10	3.7
Toscano, Lard, and Salmon	169	$4.23	3.7
Lindt's Peanut Fudge	200	$4.54	3.6
Panang Beef Curry	213	$4.45	3.6
Pepperoni Pizza Soup	177	$3.50	3.2
Peanut Cream	201	$2.01	3.2
Pepperoni Swiss Rolls	152	$6.72	3.2
Cashew Butter Butter	183	$2.55	3.2
Seaweed Maw Soup	191	$6.81	3.2
Coconut Chocolate Trailmix with Choczero 92%	187	$6.11	3.1
Cheddar, Butter, and Cherry	152	$2.75	3.1

Italian Spinach and Sausage Soup	195	$3.95	3.0
Dark Pine Trail Mix Green & Blacks 85%	202	$5.27	3.0
Almond Butter Butter	183	$2.55	3.0
Coconut Chocolate Trailmix with Green & Black's 85%	210	$5.46	3.0
Cheddar Bacon Soup	154	$5.61	2.9
Peanut Butter Butter	183	$1.67	2.9
Peanut Cream with Cacao Nibs	199	$3.31	2.9
Pork and Cabbage Soup	178	$3.58	2.9
Spicy Sesame Mushroom Soup	217	$5.93	2.8
Scrambled Eggs	186	$4.04	2.8
Thai Coconut Chicken Soup (Tom Ka Gai)	204	$4.72	2.8
Scrambled Eggs and Sausage	189	$5.92	2.5
Smoked Gouda, Butter and Apple	144	$3.38	2.4
Cheater's Hot Chocolate	166	$7.15	2.1
Split Pea Soup	188	$2.07	2.1
Machacado and Beef Tallow Pemmican	176	$10.58	1.4
Peanut Butter	166	$0.78	1.2
Trail Mix- Peanuts, Raisins, M & Ms, Almonds and Cashews	149	$1.30	0.5
Ritz Cracker Sandwiches	144	$1.86	0.4
Snicker's Bar Full Size	102	$1.65	0.3
Oreo Double Stuf	135	$1.28	0.3
Swiss Rolls (2 count)	124	$0.62	0.3
3z Glazed Honey Bun	112	$3.19	0.3
Beef Stroganoff with Noodles	128	$8.36	0.3

Instant Ramen Noodles	127	$2.00	0.2
Oats and Honey Granola Bars	127	$2.32	0.2
Goldfish	131	$1.60	0.2
Twinkies (2 count)	98	$2.15	0.2
Chili Mac with Beef	119	$8.43	0.1
Pop-Tart Frosted Strawberry (1 count)	108	$1.63	0.1
Beef Jerky- Jack Link's	80	$17.13	0.1
Fig Newtons	100	$2.29	0.1
Instant Oatmeal	100	$2.20	0.1
Easy Mac	106	$3.23	0.1
Skittles	112	$1.87	0.0
Plain Bagel- Thomas Brand	102	$1.65	0.0
Rice Sides- Chicken Rice and Pasta Blend	102	$1.65	0.0
Red Beans and Rice	98	$7.60	0.0
Swedish Fish	105	$1.99	0.0
*Classic Backpacking Foods Highlighted in Grey			

Wilder Ratio and Weight Efficiency

This chart shows the relationship between how ketogenic a food is and how efficient it is in providing calories for its weight. The chart includes the data from the same 23 classic backpacking foods as well as most of the recipes in this book. Foods with extremely high or incalculable Wilder ratios were excluded.

In the bottom left hand corner of the graph you find all the classic backpacking foods clustered together. There is a break, then the recipes in this book begin. Foods in the center tend to be high in protein. There is a slight improvement in weight efficiency with more ketogenic foods, but this varies greatly according to how much textural variety ingredients such as seaweed and mushrooms are included.

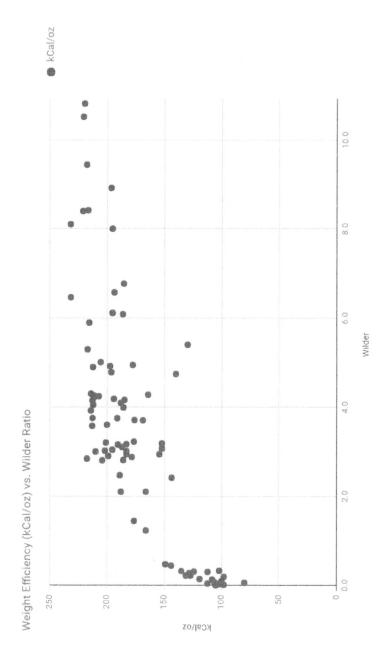

Weight Efficiency (kCal/oz) vs. Wilder Ratio

● kCal/oz

Wilder

kCal/oz

VII. REFERENCES

1. Wilson C. *What, when & water: Nutrition for weight loss wellness by clyde wilson.* ; 2007. http://www.lulu.com/shop/clyde-wilson/what-when-water-nutrition-for-weight-loss-wellness/paperback/product-1314379.html. Accessed Nov 19, 2017.

2. Volek J, Phinney S. *The art and science of low carbohydrate performance | art and science of low carb.* Beyond Obesity LLC; 2012. http://www.artandscienceoflowcarb.com/the-art-and-science-of-low-carbohydrate-performance/. Accessed Oct 12, 2017.

3. Mercola J. *Fat for fuel: A revolutionary diet to combat cancer, boost brain power, and increase your energy.* Hay House, Incorporated; 2017. Accessed Nov 7, 2017.

4. Greenfield B. *Beyond training: Mastering endurance, health & life.* Simon and Schuster; 2014. Accessed Oct 12, 2017.

5. Fung DJ. *The obesity code: Unlocking the secrets of weight loss.* Greystone Books Ltd; 2016. Accessed Dec 10, 2017.

6. Sisson M. *The primal blueprint.* Primal Nutrition; 2009. Accessed Dec 10, 2017.

7. Kresser C. *Unconventional medicine.* ; 2017.

8. Asprey D. *The bulletproof diet: Lose up to a pound a day, reclaim energy and focus, upgrade your life.* Rodale; 2014. Accessed Nov 18, 2017.

9. Moore J, MD EW. *Keto clarity: Your definitive guide to the benefits of a low-carb, high-fat diet.* Victory Belt Publishing; 2014. Accessed Dec 10, 2017.

10. Wilson J, Lowery R. *The ketogenic bible: The authoritative guide to ketosis.* Simon and Schuster; 2017. Accessed Oct 28, 2017.

11. Phinney SD, Bistrian BR, Evans WJ, Gervino E, Blackburn GL. The human metabolic response to chronic ketosis without caloric restriction: Preservation of submaximal exercise capability with reduced carbohydrate oxidation. *Metabolism.* 1983;32(8):769-776. http://www.sciencedirect.com/science/article/pii/00260495 83901063. Accessed Oct 12, 2017. doi: 10.1016/0026-0495(83)90106-3.

12. Pinckaers P, Churchward-Venne T, Bailey D, van Loon L. Ketone bodies and exercise performance: The next magic bullet or merely hype? *Sports Med.* 2017;47(3):383-391. https://search.proquest.com/docview/1924515097. doi: 10.1007/s40279-016-0577-y.

13. Noakes T, Proudfoot J, Creed S. *The real meal revolution: The radical, sustainable approach to healthy eating.* Little, Brown Book Group; 2015. Accessed Oct 12, 2017.

14. Phielix E, Szendroedi J, Roden M. Mitochondrial function and insulin resistance during aging: A mini-review. *Gerontology.* 2011;57(5):387-396. Accessed Oct 28, 2017. doi: 10.1159/000317691.

15. Ioannou GN, Bryson CL, Boyko EJ. Prevalence and trends of insulin resistance, impaired fasting glucose, and diabetes. *Journal of Diabetes and its Complications.* 2007;21(6):363-370. http://www.sciencedirect.com/science/article/pii/S1056872 706000766. Accessed Oct 12, 2017. doi: 10.1016/j.jdiacomp.2006.07.005.

16. Sidossis LS, Stuart CA, Shulman GI, Lopaschuk GD, Wolfe RR. Glucose plus insulin regulate fat oxidation by controlling the rate of fatty acid entry into the mitochondria. *The Journal of clinical investigation.* 1996;98(10):2244-2250. http://www.ncbi.nlm.nih.gov/pubmed/8941640. doi: 10.1172/JCI119034.

17. Rydén M, Jocken J, van Harmelen V, et al. Comparative studies of the role of hormone-sensitive lipase and adipose triglyceride lipase in human fat cell lipolysis. *Am J Physiol Endocrinol Metab.* 2007;292(6):1847. Accessed Oct 28, 2017. doi: 10.1152/ajpendo.00040.2007.

18. Cornier M, Donahoo WT, Pereira R, et al. Insulin sensitivity determines the effectiveness of dietary macronutrient composition on weight loss in obese women. *Obes Res.* 2005;13(4):703-709. Accessed Nov 5, 2017. doi: 10.1038/oby.2005.79.

19. Volek JS, Quann EE, Forsythe CE. Low-carbohydrate diets promote a more favorable body composition than low-fat diets. *Strength & Conditioning Journal.* 2010;32(1):42–47. http://journals.lww.com/nsca-scj/Abstract/2010/02000/Low_Carbohydrate_Diets_Promote_a_More_Favorable.6.aspx. Accessed Oct 12, 2017. doi: 10.1519/SSC.0b013e3181c16c41.

20. Young CM, Scanlan SS, Im HS, Lutwak L. Effect of body composition and other parameters in obese young men of carbohydrate level of reduction diet. *Am J Clin Nutr.* 1971;24(3):290-296. Accessed Oct 28, 2017.

21. Sherwin RS, Hendler RG, Felig P. Effect of ketone infusions on amino acid and nitrogen metabolism in man. *J Clin Invest.* 1975;55(6):1382-1390. Accessed Oct 28, 2017. doi: 10.1172/JCI108057.

22. Palaiologos G, Felig P. Effects of ketone bodies on amino acid metabolism in isolated rat diaphragm. *Biochem J*. 1976;154(3):709-716. Accessed Oct 28, 2017.

23. Dieter BP, Schoenfeld BJ, Aragon AA. The data do not seem to support a benefit to BCAA supplementation during periods of caloric restriction. *J Int Soc Sports Nutr*. 2016;13:21. Accessed Nov 19, 2017. doi: 10.1186/s12970-016-0128-9.

24. Dudgeon WD, Kelley EP, Scheett TP. In a single-blind, matched group design: Branched-chain amino acid supplementation and resistance training maintains lean body mass during a caloric restricted diet. *J Int Soc Sports Nutr*. 2016;13:1. Accessed Nov 19, 2017. doi: 10.1186/s12970-015-0112-9.

25. Gregory R. A low-carbohydrate ketogenic diet combined with 6 weeks of crossfit training improves body composition and performance. *Masters Theses*. 2016. http://commons.lib.jmu.edu/master201019/109. Accessed Nov 19, 2017.

26. Ainsworth BE, Haskell WL, Herrmann SD, et al. 2011 compendium of physical activities: A second update of codes and MET values. *Med Sci Sports Exerc*. 2011;43(8):1575-1581. Accessed Oct 28, 2017. doi: 10.1249/MSS.0b013e31821ece12.

27. Forsythe CE, Phinney SD, Fernandez ML, et al. Comparison of low fat and low carbohydrate diets on circulating fatty acid composition and markers of inflammation. *Lipids*. 2008;43(1):65-77. Accessed Oct 28, 2017. doi: 10.1007/s11745-007-3132-7.

28. Kim DY, Davis LM, Sullivan PG, et al. Ketone bodies are protective against oxidative stress in neocortical

neurons. *J Neurochem*. 2007;101(5):1316-1326. Accessed Oct 28, 2017. doi: 10.1111/j.1471-4159.2007.04483.x.

29. Maalouf M, Sullivan PG, Davis L, Kim DY, Rho JM. Ketones inhibit mitochondrial production of reactive oxygen species production following glutamate excitotoxicity by increasing NADH oxidation. *Neuroscience*. 2007;145(1):256-264. Accessed Oct 28, 2017. doi: 10.1016/j.neuroscience.2006.11.065.

30. Nazarewicz RR, Ziolkowski W, Vaccaro PS, Ghafourifar P. Effect of short-term ketogenic diet on redox status of human blood. *Rejuvenation Res*. 2007;10(4):435-440. Accessed Nov 16, 2017. doi: 10.1089/rej.2007.0540.

31. Rhyu H, Cho S, Roh H. The effects of ketogenic diet on oxidative stress and antioxidative capacity markers of taekwondo athletes. *JER*. 2014;10(6):362-366. http://www.earticle.net/Article.aspx?sn=238381. doi: 10.12965/jer.140178.

32. Milder JB, Patel M. Modulation of oxidative stress and mitochondrial function by the ketogenic diet. *Epilepsy Res*. 2012;100(3):295-303. https://www.ncbi.nlm.nih.gov/pmc/articles/PMC3322307/. Accessed Oct 28, 2017. doi: 10.1016/j.eplepsyres.2011.09.021.

33. Blundell JE, Burley VJ, Cotton JR, Lawton CL. Dietary fat and the control of energy intake: Evaluating the effects of fat on meal size and postmeal satiety. *Am J Clin Nutr*. 1993;57(5 Suppl):778S. Accessed Oct 28, 2017.

34. Samra RA. Fats and satiety. In: Montmayeur J, le Coutre J, eds. *Fat detection: Taste, texture, and post ingestive effects*. Boca Raton (FL): CRC Press/Taylor & Francis; 2010.

http://www.ncbi.nlm.nih.gov/books/NBK53550/. Accessed
Oct 28, 2017.

35. Gibson AA, Seimon RV, Lee CMY, et al. Do ketogenic
diets really suppress appetite? A systematic review and
meta-analysis. *Obesity Reviews*. 2015;16(1):64-76.
http://onlinelibrary.wiley.com/doi/10.1111/obr.12230/abstr
act. doi: 10.1111/obr.12230.

36. Heini AF, Kirk KA, Lara-Castro C, Weinsier RL.
Relationship between hunger-satiety feelings and various
metabolic parameters in women with obesity during
controlled weight loss. *Obesity research*. 1998;6(3):225-
230. http://www.ncbi.nlm.nih.gov/pubmed/9618127. doi:
10.1002/j.1550-8528.1998.tb00341.x.

37. Slavin J, Green H. Dietary fibre and satiety. *Nutrition
Bulletin*. 2007;32(s1):32-42.
http://onlinelibrary.wiley.com/doi/10.1111/j.1467-
3010.2007.00603.x/abstract. doi: 10.1111/j.1467-
3010.2007.00603.x.

38. Wang IX, Ramrattan G, Cheung VG. Genetic variation
in insulin-induced kinase signaling. *Mol Syst Biol*.
2015;11(7):820. Accessed Oct 28, 2017.

39. Leino RL, Gerhart DZ, Duelli R, Enerson BE, Drewes
LR. Diet-induced ketosis increases monocarboxylate
transporter (MCT1) levels in rat brain. *Neurochem Int*.
2001;38(6):519-527. Accessed Oct 28, 2017.

40. Hall JE. *Guyton and hall textbook of medical
physiology E-book*. Elsevier Health Sciences; 2015.
Accessed Oct 28, 2017.

41. Grabacka M, Pierzchalska M, Dean M, Reiss K.
Regulation of ketone body metabolism and the role of

PPARα. *International Journal of Molecular Sciences.*
2016;17(12):2093.
https://doaj.org/article/0ea07dae22214ae5becd64db7c2558
05. doi: 10.3390/ijms17122093.

42. Baba H, Zhang XJ, Wolfe RR. Glycerol
gluconeogenesis in fasting humans. *Nutrition.*
1995;11(2):149-153. Accessed Oct 28, 2017.

43. Bougneres PF, Lemmel C, Ferré P, Bier DM. Abstract.
Abstract. 1986;77(1):42-48.
https://www.ncbi.nlm.nih.gov/pmc/articles/PMC423306/.

44. Insel PM, Ross D, McMahon K. *Nutrition.* Jones &
Bartlett Learning; 2013. Accessed Nov 2, 2017.

45. Pogozelski W, Arpaia N, Priore S. The metabolic
effects of low-carbohydrate diets and incorporation into a
biochemistry course. *Biochemistry and molecular biology
education : a bimonthly publication of the International
Union of Biochemistry and Molecular Biology.*
2005;33(2):91-100.
http://www.ncbi.nlm.nih.gov/pubmed/21638552. doi:
10.1002/bmb.2005.494033022445.

46. Adam-Perrot A, Clifton P, Brouns F. Low-carbohydrate
diets: Nutritional and physiological aspects. *Obes Rev.*
2006;7(1):49-58. Accessed Oct 28, 2017. doi:
10.1111/j.1467-789X.2006.00222.x.

47. Alberti KG, Johnston DG, Gill A, Barnes AJ, Orskov
H. Hormonal regulation of ketone-body metabolism in
man. *Biochem Soc Symp.* 1978(43):163-182. Accessed Oct
28, 2017.

48. Susanne HA Holt, Janette C Brand Miller, Peter Petocz.
Aninsulinindexoffoods:Theinsulindemandgeneratedby. *Am*

J Clin Nutr. 1997;66(5):1264-1276.
http://ajcn.nutrition.org/content/66/5/1264. Accessed Oct 12, 2017.

49. Streja DA, Marliss EB, Steiner G. The effects of prolonged fasting on plasma triglyceride kinetics in man. *Metabolism*. 1977;26(5):505-516.
http://www.sciencedirect.com/science/article/pii/00260495 77900944. Accessed Oct 28, 2017. doi: 10.1016/0026-0495(77)90094-4.

50. Cahill GF. Fuel metabolism in starvation. *Annu Rev Nutr*. 2006;26:1-22. Accessed Oct 28, 2017. doi: 10.1146/annurev.nutr.26.061505.111258.

51. Gleeson M, Greenhaff PL, Maughan RJ. Influence of a 24 h fast on high intensity cycle exercise performance in man. *European journal of applied physiology and occupational physiology*. 1988;57(6):653-659.
http://www.ncbi.nlm.nih.gov/pubmed/3416848. doi: 10.1007/BF01075984.

52. Harvie MN, Pegington M, Mattson MP, et al. The effects of intermittent or continuous energy restriction on weight loss and metabolic disease risk markers: A randomized trial in young overweight women. *International Journal of Obesity*. 2011;35(5):714-727.
http://dx.doi.org/10.1038/ijo.2010.171. doi: 10.1038/ijo.2010.171.

53. Catenacci VA, Pan Z, Ostendorf D, et al. A randomized pilot study comparing zero-calorie alternate-day fasting to daily caloric restriction in adults with obesity. *Obesity*. 2016;24(9):1874-1883.
http://onlinelibrary.wiley.com/doi/10.1002/oby.21581/abstr act. doi: 10.1002/oby.21581.

54. Ross BD, Hems R, Krebs HA. The rate of gluconeogenesis from various precursors in the perfused rat liver. *Biochem J*. 1967;102(3):942-951. Accessed Oct 28, 2017.

55. Yoshiharu Shimomura, Taro Murakami, Naoya Nakai, Masaru Nagasaki, Robert A Harris. Exercise promotes BCAA catabolism: Effects of BCAA supplementation on skeletal muscle during Exercise1. *The Journal of Nutrition*. 2004;134(6S):1583S. https://search.proquest.com/docview/197447484.

56. Feo PD, Loreto CD, Lucidi P, et al. Metabolic response to exercise. *J Endocrinol Invest*. 2003;26(9):851-854. https://link.springer.com/article/10.1007/BF03345235. Accessed Nov 2, 2017. doi: 10.1007/BF03345235.

57. Manninen AH. Very-low-carbohydrate diets and preservation of muscle mass. *Nutrition & metabolism*. 2006;3(1):9. http://www.ncbi.nlm.nih.gov/pubmed/16448570. doi: 10.1186/1743-7075-3-9.

58. Heymsfield SB, Gonzalez MCC, Shen W, Redman L, Thomas D. Weight loss composition is one-fourth fat-free mass: A critical review and critique of this widely cited rule. *Obes Rev*. 2014;15(4):310-321. Accessed Nov 19, 2017. doi: 10.1111/obr.12143.

59. Moreno B, Bellido D, Sajoux I, et al. Comparison of a very low-calorie-ketogenic diet with a standard low-calorie diet in the treatment of obesity. *Endocrine*. 2014;47(3):793-805. Accessed Nov 19, 2017. doi: 10.1007/s12020-014-0192-3.

60. Noakes M, Foster PR, Keogh JB, James AP, Mamo JC, Clifton PM. Comparison of isocaloric very low

carbohydrate/high saturated fat and high carbohydrate/low saturated fat diets on body composition and cardiovascular risk. *Nutr Metab (Lond)*. 2006;3:7. Accessed Nov 19, 2017. doi: 10.1186/1743-7075-3-7.

61. Volek J, Sharman M, Gómez A, et al. Comparison of energy-restricted very low-carbohydrate and low-fat diets on weight loss and body composition in overweight men and women. *Nutr Metab (Lond)*. 2004;1(1):13. Accessed Nov 19, 2017. doi: 10.1186/1743-7075-1-13.

62. Krieger JW, Sitren HS, Daniels MJ, Langkamp-Henken B. Effects of variation in protein and carbohydrate intake on body mass and composition during energy restriction: A meta-regression 1. *Am J Clin Nutr*. 2006;83(2):260-274. Accessed Nov 19, 2017.

63. Manninen AH. Very-low-carbohydrate diets and preservation of muscle mass. *Nutrition & metabolism*. 2006;3(1):9. http://www.ncbi.nlm.nih.gov/pubmed/16448570. doi: 10.1186/1743-7075-3-9.

64. V Issurin. Duration and practical components of the residual effects of training. *LG Classification Performance Port*. 2004.

65. Kahlhöfer J, Lagerpusch M, Enderle J, et al. Carbohydrate intake and glycemic index affect substrate oxidation during a controlled weight cycle in healthy men. *Eur J Clin Nutr*. 2014;68(9):1060-1066. Accessed Nov 5, 2017. doi: 10.1038/ejcn.2014.132.

66. Isken F, Klaus S, Petzke KJ, Loddenkemper C, Pfeiffer AFH, Weickert MO. Impairment of fat oxidation under high- vs. low-glycemic index diet occurs before the development of an obese phenotype. *Am J Physiol*

Endocrinol Metab. 2010;298(2):287. Accessed Nov 5, 2017. doi: 10.1152/ajpendo.00515.2009.

67. Simopoulos AP. Evolutionary aspects of the dietary omega-6/omega-3 fatty acid ratio: Medical implications. In: *Evolutionary thinking in medicine.* Springer, Cham; 2016:119-134. https://link.springer.com/chapter/10.1007/978-3-319-29716-3_9. Accessed Nov 2, 2017.

68. Simopoulos AP. An increase in the omega-6/omega-3 fatty acid ratio increases the risk for obesity. *Nutrients.* 2016;8(3):128. http://www.ncbi.nlm.nih.gov/pubmed/26950145. doi: 10.3390/nu8030128.

69. Ashwar BA, Gani A, Shah A, Wani IA, Masoodi FA. Preparation, health benefits and applications of resistant starch—a review. *Starch - Stärke.* 2016;68(3-4):287-301. http://onlinelibrary.wiley.com/doi/10.1002/star.201500064/abstract. doi: 10.1002/star.201500064.

70. Desmarchelier C, Ludwig T, Scheundel R, et al. Diet-induced obesity in ad libitum-fed mice: Food texture overrides the effect of macronutrient composition. *British Journal of Nutrition.* 2013;109(8):1518-1527. https://www.cambridge.org/core/journals/british-journal-of-nutrition/article/diet-induced-obesity-in-ad-libitum-fed-mice-food-texture-overrides-the-effect-of-macronutrient-composition/725D71275CF7399332CEC8C9C76BE23F. Accessed Nov 5, 2017. doi: 10.1017/S0007114512003340.

71. Wong JMW, Jenkins DJA. Carbohydrate digestibility and metabolic effects. *J Nutr.* 2007;137(11):2546S. http://jn.nutrition.org/content/137/11/2539S. Accessed Nov 2, 2017.

72. Melsom T, Schei J, Stefansson VTN, et al. Prediabetes and risk of glomerular hyperfiltration and albuminuria in the general nondiabetic population: A prospective cohort study. *American Journal of Kidney Diseases.* 2016;67(6):841-850. http://www.sciencedirect.com/science/article/pii/S0272638 61501389X. doi: 10.1053/j.ajkd.2015.10.025.

73. Grundy SM. Pre-diabetes, metabolic syndrome, and cardiovascular risk. *J Am Coll Cardiol.* 2012;59(7):635-643. Accessed Nov 5, 2017. doi: 10.1016/j.jacc.2011.08.080.

74. Sasazuki S, Charvat H, Hara A, et al. Diabetes mellitus and cancer risk: Pooled analysis of eight cohort studies in japan. *Cancer Sci.* 2013;104(11):1499-1507. Accessed Nov 5, 2017. doi: 10.1111/cas.12241.

75. Huang Y, Cai X, Qiu M, et al. Prediabetes and the risk of cancer: A meta-analysis. *Diabetologia.* 2014;57(11):2261-2269. Accessed Nov 5, 2017. doi: 10.1007/s00125-014-3361-2.

76. Mirmiran P, Tohidi M, Bahadoran Z, Azizi F, Esfandiari S. Dietary insulin load and insulin index are associated with the risk of insulin resistance: A prospective approach in tehran lipid and glucose study. *Journal of Diabetes and Metabolic Disorders.* 2016;15(1). https://search.proquest.com/docview/1807951524. doi: 10.1186/s40200-016-0247-5.

77. Hollenbeck CB, Chen N, Chen YD, Reaven GM. Relationship between the plasma insulin response to oral glucose and insulin-stimulated glucose utilization in normal subjects. *Diabetes.* 1984;33(5):460-463. Accessed Nov 5, 2017.

78. Martínez-Fernández L, Laiglesia LM, Huerta AE, Martínez JA, Moreno-Aliaga MJ. Omega-3 fatty acids and adipose tissue function in obesity and metabolic syndrome. *Prostaglandins Other Lipid Mediat*. 2015;121(Pt A):24-41. Accessed Nov 5, 2017. doi: 10.1016/j.prostaglandins.2015.07.003.

79. Karst K. *The metabolic syndrome program: How to lose weight, beat heart disease, stop insulin resistance and more*. John Wiley & Sons; 2008. Accessed Nov 5, 2017.

80. Schönfeld P, Wojtczak L. Short- and medium-chain fatty acids in energy metabolism: The cellular perspective. *J Lipid Res*. 2016;57(6):943-954. Accessed Nov 7, 2017. doi: 10.1194/jlr.R067629.

81. Liu YC, Wang H. Medium-chain triglyceride ketogenic diet, an effective treatment for drug-resistant epilepsy and a comparison with other ketogenic diets. *Biomed J*. 2013;36(1):9-15. Accessed Nov 7, 2017. doi: 10.4103/2319-4170.107154.

82. Otles S, Ozgoz S. Health effects of dietary fiber. *Acta Sci Pol Technol Aliment*. 2014;13(2):191-202. Accessed Nov 7, 2017.

83. Jenkins DJ, Kendall CW, Vuksan V. Viscous fibers, health claims, and strategies to reduce cardiovascular disease risk. *Am J Clin Nutr*. 2000;71(2):401-402. http://ajcn.nutrition.org/content/71/2/401. Accessed Nov 7, 2017.

84. Festi D, Schiumerini R, Eusebi LH, Marasco G, Taddia M, Colecchia A. Gut microbiota and metabolic syndrome. *World J Gastroenterol*. 2014;20(43):16079-16094. Accessed Nov 7, 2017. doi: 10.3748/wjg.v20.i43.16079.

85. Raigond P, Ezekiel R, Raigond B. Resistant starch in food: A review. *J Sci Food Agric*. 2015;95(10):1968-1978. Accessed Nov 7, 2017. doi: 10.1002/jsfa.6966.

86. Bindels LB, Walter J, Ramer-Tait AE. Resistant starches for the management of metabolic diseases. *Curr Opin Clin Nutr Metab Care*. 2015;18(6):559-565. Accessed Nov 7, 2017. doi: 10.1097/MCO.0000000000000223.

87. Keenan MJ, Zhou J, Hegsted M, et al. Role of resistant starch in improving gut health, adiposity, and insulin resistance. *Adv Nutr*. 2015;6(2):198-205. Accessed Nov 7, 2017. doi: 10.3945/an.114.007419.

88. Higgins JA, Higbee DR, Donahoo WT, Brown IL, Bell ML, Bessesen DH. Resistant starch consumption promotes lipid oxidation. *Nutr Metab (Lond)*. 2004;1(1):8. Accessed Nov 7, 2017. doi: 10.1186/1743-7075-1-8.

89. Robertson MD, Bickerton AS, Dennis AL, Vidal H, Frayn KN. Insulin-sensitizing effects of dietary resistant starch and effects on skeletal muscle and adipose tissue metabolism. *Am J Clin Nutr*. 2005;82(3):559-567. Accessed Nov 7, 2017.

90. Johnston KL, Thomas EL, Bell JD, Frost GS, Robertson MD. Resistant starch improves insulin sensitivity in metabolic syndrome. *Diabetic Medicine*. 2010;27(4):391-397. http://onlinelibrary.wiley.com/doi/10.1111/j.1464-5491.2010.02923.x/abstract. Accessed Nov 7, 2017. doi: 10.1111/j.1464-5491.2010.02923.x.

91. Ebbeling CB, Leidig MM, Feldman HA, Lovesky MM, Ludwig DS. Effects of a low-glycemic load vs low-fat diet in obese young adults: A randomized trial. *JAMA*.

2007;297(19):2092-2102. Accessed Nov 5, 2017. doi:
10.1001/jama.297.19.2092.

92. World Health Organization, Food and Agriculture
Organization of the United Nations, United Nations
University. Protein and amino acid requirements in human
nutrition. report of a joint FAO/WHO/UNU expert
consultation. *WHO*. 2007.
http://www.who.int/nutrition/publications/nutrientrequirem
ents/WHO_TRS_935/en/. Accessed Nov 7, 2017.

93. Board, Institute of Medicine (US) Food and Nutrition.
What are dietary reference intakes? National Academies
Press (US); 1998.
https://www.ncbi.nlm.nih.gov/books/NBK45182/.
Accessed Nov 18, 2017.

94. Fung J. *The obesity code: Unlocking the secrets of
weight loss.* Greystone Books; 2016. Accessed Nov 7,
2017.

95. Harnack LJ, Jeffery RW, Boutelle KN. Temporal trends
in energy intake in the united states: An ecologic
perspective. *Am J Clin Nutr*. 2000;71(6):1478-1484.
Accessed Nov 7, 2017.

96. Howard BV, Manson JE, Stefanick ML, et al. Low-fat
dietary pattern and weight change over 7 years: The
women's health initiative dietary modification trial. *JAMA*.
2006;295(1):39-49. Accessed Nov 7, 2017. doi:
10.1001/jama.295.1.39.

97. Howard BV, Van Horn L, Hsia J, et al. Low-fat dietary
pattern and risk of cardiovascular disease: The women's
health initiative randomized controlled dietary modification
trial. *JAMA*. 2006;295(6):655-666. Accessed Nov 7, 2017.
doi: 10.1001/jama.295.6.655.

98. Beresford SAA, Johnson KC, Ritenbaugh C, et al. Low-fat dietary pattern and risk of colorectal cancer: The women's health initiative randomized controlled dietary modification trial. *JAMA*. 2006;295(6):643-654. Accessed Nov 7, 2017. doi: 10.1001/jama.295.6.643.

99. Prentice RL, Caan B, Chlebowski RT, et al. Low-fat dietary pattern and risk of invasive breast cancer: The women's health initiative randomized controlled dietary modification trial. *JAMA*. 2006;295(6):629-642. Accessed Nov 7, 2017. doi: 10.1001/jama.295.6.629.

100. Kapetanakis M, Liuba P, Odermarsky M, Lundgren J, Hallböök T. Effects of ketogenic diet on vascular function. *Eur J Paediatr Neurol*. 2014;18(4):489-494. Accessed Nov 9, 2017. doi: 10.1016/j.ejpn.2014.03.006.

101. Bueno NB, de Melo, Ingrid Sofia Vieira, de Oliveira SL, da Rocha Ataide T. Very-low-carbohydrate ketogenic diet v. low-fat diet for long-term weight loss: A meta-analysis of randomised controlled trials. *Br J Nutr*. 2013;110(7):1178-1187. Accessed Nov 9, 2017. doi: 10.1017/S0007114513000548.

102. Yancy WS, Olsen MK, Guyton JR, Bakst RP, Westman EC. A low-carbohydrate, ketogenic diet versus a low-fat diet to treat obesity and hyperlipidemia: A randomized, controlled trial. *Ann Intern Med*. 2004;140(10):769-777. Accessed Nov 13, 2017.

103. Moore KJ, Sheedy FJ, Fisher EA. Macrophages in atherosclerosis: A dynamic balance. *Nature Reviews Immunology*. 2013;13(10):nri3520. https://www.nature.com/articles/nri3520. Accessed Nov 11, 2017. doi: 10.1038/nri3520.

104. Volek J, MD, Phd Stephen D Phinney, Phd, Rd Jeff S Volek, Phinney SD. *The art and science of low carbohydrate living: An expert guide to making the life-saving benefits of carbohydrate restriction sustainable and enjoyable.* Beyond Obesity; 2011. Accessed Oct 12, 2017.

105. Rankin JW, Turpyn AD. Low carbohydrate, high fat diet increases C-reactive protein during weight loss. *J Am Coll Nutr.* 2007;26(2):163-169. Accessed Nov 9, 2017.

106. Noto H, Goto A, Tsujimoto T, Noda M. Low-carbohydrate diets and all-cause mortality: A systematic review and meta-analysis of observational studies. *PLoS ONE.* 2013;8(1):e55030. Accessed Nov 9, 2017. doi: 10.1371/journal.pone.0055030.

107. Seneff S, Wainwright G, Mascitelli L. Nutrition and alzheimer's disease: The detrimental role of a high carbohydrate diet. *European Journal of Internal Medicine.* 2011;22(2):134-140. http://www.ejinme.com/article/S0953-6205(11)00004-5/fulltext. Accessed Nov 11, 2017. doi: 10.1016/j.ejim.2010.12.017.

108. Neuhouser M, Lichtensein A, Abrams S, Anderson C, Story M, Millen B. Science base chapter:
Food and nutrient intakes,
and health:
Current status and trends *Dietary Guidelines Advisory Committee.* 2014:1-40.

109. Lichtenstein AH. Dietary trans fatty acids and cardiovascular disease risk: Past and present. *Curr Atheroscler Rep.* 2014;16(8):433. Accessed Nov 7, 2017. doi: 10.1007/s11883-014-0433-1.

110. Bendsen NT, Stender S, Szecsi PB, et al. Effect of industrially produced trans fat on markers of systemic

inflammation: Evidence from a randomized trial in women. *J Lipid Res*. 2011;52(10):1821-1828. Accessed Nov 9, 2017. doi: 10.1194/jlr.M014738.

111. Chowdhury R, Warnakula S, Kunutsor S, et al. Association of dietary, circulating, and supplement fatty acids with coronary risk: A systematic review and meta-analysis. *Ann Intern Med*. 2014;160(6):398-406. Accessed Nov 7, 2017. doi: 10.7326/M13-1788.

112. Ramsden CE, Zamora D, Leelarthaepin B, et al. Use of dietary linoleic acid for secondary prevention of coronary heart disease and death: Evaluation of recovered data from the sydney diet heart study and updated meta-analysis. *BMJ*. 2013;346:e8707. Accessed Nov 11, 2017.

113. Superko HR, Superko AR, Lundberg GP, et al. Omega-3 fatty acid blood levels clinical significance update. *Curr Cardiovasc Risk Rep*. 2014;8(11):407. Accessed Nov 9, 2017. doi: 10.1007/s12170-014-0407-4.

114. Howe P, Buckley J. Metabolic health benefits of long-chain omega-3 polyunsaturated fatty acids. *Mil Med*. 2014;179(11 Suppl):138-143. Accessed Nov 11, 2017. doi: 10.7205/MILMED-D-14-00154.

115. Lane K, Derbyshire E, Li W, Brennan C. Bioavailability and potential uses of vegetarian sources of omega-3 fatty acids: A review of the literature. *Crit Rev Food Sci Nutr*. 2014;54(5):572-579. Accessed Nov 11, 2017. doi: 10.1080/10408398.2011.596292.

116. Vieira SA, Zhang G, Decker EA. Biological implications of lipid oxidation products. *J Am Oil Chem Soc*. 2017;94(3):339-351. https://link.springer.com/article/10.1007/s11746-017-2958-

2. Accessed Nov 11, 2017. doi: 10.1007/s11746-017-2958-2.

117. Frankel EN. *Lipid oxidation.* Elsevier; 2014. Accessed Nov 11, 2017.

118. Delgado C, Guinard J. How do consumer hedonic ratings for extra virgin olive oil relate to quality ratings by experts and descriptive analysis ratings? *Food Quality and Preference.* 2011;22(2):213-225. http://www.sciencedirect.com/science/article/pii/S0950329310001977. Accessed Nov 11, 2017. doi: 10.1016/j.foodqual.2010.10.004.

119. Monteleone E, Langstaff S. *Olive oil sensory science.* John Wiley & Sons; 2013. Accessed Nov 11, 2017.

120. Frankel E, Mailer R, Shoemaker C, Wang S, Flynn D. Tests indicate that imported "extra virgin"olive oil often fails
international and USDA standards. *UC Davis Olive Center.* 2010.

121. Deatherage F. *Food for life.* Springer Science & Business Media; 2013. Accessed Nov 11, 2017.

122. Halliwell B, Zhao K, Whiteman M. The gastrointestinal tract: A major site of antioxidant action? *Free Radic Res.* 2000;33(6):819-830. Accessed Nov 11, 2017.

123. Toufektsian M, Salen P, Laporte F, Tonelli C, de Lorgeril M. Dietary flavonoids increase plasma very long-chain (n-3) fatty acids in rats. *J Nutr.* 2011;141(1):37-41. Accessed Nov 11, 2017. doi: 10.3945/jn.110.127225.

124. Campbell TC, (II.) TMC. *The china study: The most comprehensive study of nutrition ever conducted and the startling implications for diet, weight loss and long-term health.* BenBella Books; 2006. Accessed Nov 11, 2017.

125. Milo R, Phillips R, Orme N. *Cell biology by the numbers.* New York: Garland Science; 2016.

126. Young VR, Pellett PL. Plant proteins in relation to human protein and amino acid nutrition. *Am J Clin Nutr.* 1994;59(5 Suppl):1212S. Accessed Nov 11, 2017.

127. Effect of feeding systems on omega-3 fatty acids, conjugated linoleic acid and trans fatty acids in australian beef cuts: Potential impact on human health - ProQuest. https://search.proquest.com/openview/34c8d8be10ea9a2ba 5e199ca801967cf/1?pq-origsite=gscholar&cbl=45812. Accessed Nov 2, 2017.

128. gladsby p. The inuit paradox | DiscoverMagazine.com. *Discover Magazine.* . http://discovermagazine.com/2004/oct/inuit-paradox. Accessed Nov 11, 2017.

129. Hedrén E, Diaz V, Svanberg U. Estimation of carotenoid accessibility from carrots determined by an in vitro digestion method. *Eur J Clin Nutr.* 2002;56(5):425-430. Accessed Nov 13, 2017. doi: 10.1038/sj.ejcn.1601329.

130. United States Department of Agriculture Agricultural Research Service. USDA food composition databases. . Updated 2015.

131. MALEKINEJAD H, REZABAKHSH A. Hormones in dairy foods and their impact on public health - A narrative review article. *Iran J Public Health.* 2015;44(6):742-758.

https://www.ncbi.nlm.nih.gov/pmc/articles/PMC4524299/.
Accessed Nov 11, 2017.

132. Ganmaa D, Li XM, Qin LQ, Wang PY, Takeda M,
Sato A. The experience of japan as a clue to the etiology of
testicular and prostatic cancers. *Med Hypotheses.*
2003;60(5):724-730. Accessed Nov 11, 2017.

133. Pettersson A, Kasperzyk JL, Kenfield SA, et al. Milk
and dairy consumption among men with prostate cancer
and risk of metastases and prostate cancer death. *Cancer
Epidemiol Biomarkers Prev.* 2012;21(3):428-436.
https://www.ncbi.nlm.nih.gov/pmc/articles/PMC3297731/.
Accessed Nov 11, 2017. doi: 10.1158/1055-9965.EPI-11-
1004.

134. Rautiainen S, Wang L, Lee I-, Manson JE, Buring JE,
Sesso HD. Dairy consumption in association with weight
change and risk of becoming overweight or obese in
middle-aged and older women: A prospective cohort study.
Am J Clin Nutr. 2016;103(4):979-988. Accessed Nov 11,
2017. doi: 10.3945/ajcn.115.118406.

135. Food Allergy Research and Education. Food allergy
facts and statistics for the U.S. .

136. de Verdier MG, Hagman U, Peters RK, Steineck G,
Övervik E. Meat, cooking methods and colorectal cancer:
A case-referent study in stockholm. *Int J Cancer.*
1991;49(4):520-525.
http://onlinelibrary.wiley.com/doi/10.1002/ijc.2910490408/
abstract. Accessed Nov 11, 2017. doi:
10.1002/ijc.2910490408.

137. Muscat JE, Wynder EL. The consumption of well-
done red meat and the risk of colorectal cancer. *Am J
Public Health.* 1994;84(5):856-858.

http://ajph.aphapublications.org/doi/abs/10.2105/AJPH.84.
5.856. Accessed Nov 11, 2017. doi:
10.2105/AJPH.84.5.856.

138. Alaejos MS, González V, Afonso AM. Exposure to
heterocyclic aromatic amines from the consumption of
cooked red meat and its effect on human cancer risk: A
review. *Food Additives & Contaminants: Part A.*
2008;25(1):2-24.
http://dx.doi.org/10.1080/02652030701474235. Accessed
Nov 11, 2017. doi: 10.1080/02652030701474235.

139. Norat T, Lukanova A, Ferrari P, Riboli E. Meat
consumption and colorectal cancer risk: Dose-response
meta-analysis of epidemiological studies. *Int J Cancer.*
2002;98(2):241-256.
http://onlinelibrary.wiley.com/doi/10.1002/ijc.10126/abstra
ct. Accessed Nov 11, 2017. doi: 10.1002/ijc.10126.

140. Urquhart JA. The most northerly practice in canada.
1935. *CMAJ.* 1992;147(8):1193-1196. Accessed Dec 9,
2017.

141. Scientific American. How does mercury get into fish?
https://www.scientificamerican.com/article/how-does-
mercury-get-into/. Updated 2011. Accessed Nov 12, 2017.

142. Hassett-Sipple B, Swartout J, Schoeny R. Mercury
study report to congress. volume 5. health effects of
mercury and mercury compounds. . 1997.

143. Mahaffey KR, Clickner RP, Jeffries RA. Adult
women's blood mercury concentrations vary regionally in
the united states: Association with patterns of fish
consumption (NHANES 1999-2004). *Environ Health
Perspect.* 2009;117(1):47-53. Accessed Nov 12, 2017. doi:
10.1289/ehp.11674.

144. National Resources Defense Council. Mercury in fish. . 2006.

145. Diamond J. *The world until yesterday: What can we learn from traditional societies?* Penguin; 2012. Accessed Nov 13, 2017.

146. Ohtsuka R, Suzuki T, Morita M. Sodium-rich tree ash as a native salt source in lowland papua. *Econ Bot.* 1987;41(1):55-59. https://link.springer.com/article/10.1007/BF02859348. Accessed Nov 13, 2017. doi: 10.1007/BF02859348.

147. Montain SJ, Sawka MN, Wenger CB. Hyponatremia associated with exercise: Risk factors and pathogenesis. *Exercise and Sport Sciences Reviews.* 2001;29(3):113–117. http://journals.lww.com/acsm-essr/Abstract/2001/07000/Hyponatremia_Associated_With_Exercise__Risk.5.aspx. Accessed Nov 13, 2017.

148. CDC. Sodium and the dietary guidelines. *US Centers for Disease Control.* 2015.

149. Shin SJ, Lim C, Oh SW, Rhee M. The unique response of renin and aldosterone to dietary sodium intervention in sodium sensitivity. *J Renin Angiotensin Aldosterone Syst.* 2014;15(2):117-123. Accessed Nov 13, 2017. doi: 10.1177/1470320314526437.

150. Sharma S, McFann K, Chonchol M, Kendrick J. Dietary sodium and potassium intake is not associated with elevated blood pressure in US adults with no prior history of hypertension. *J Clin Hypertens (Greenwich).* 2014;16(6):418-423. Accessed Nov 13, 2017. doi: 10.1111/jch.12312.

151. Farquhar WB, Edwards DG, Jurkovitz CT, Weintraub WS. Dietary sodium and health: More than just blood pressure. *J Am Coll Cardiol.* 2015;65(10):1042-1050. Accessed Nov 13, 2017. doi: 10.1016/j.jacc.2014.12.039.

152. Cook NR, Obarzanek E, Cutler JA, et al. Joint effects of sodium and potassium intake on subsequent cardiovascular disease: The trials of hypertension prevention follow-up study. *Arch Intern Med.* 2009;169(1):32-40. Accessed Nov 16, 2017. doi: 10.1001/archinternmed.2008.523.

153. Clegg ME, McKenna P, McClean C, et al. Gastrointestinal transit, post-prandial lipaemia and satiety following 3 days high-fat diet in men. *Eur J Clin Nutr.* 2011;65(2):240-246. Accessed Nov 16, 2017. doi: 10.1038/ejcn.2010.235.

154. Cunningham KM, Daly J, Horowitz M, Read NW. Gastrointestinal adaptation to diets of differing fat composition in human volunteers. *Gut.* 1991;32(5):483-486. Accessed Nov 16, 2017.

155. Maldonado-Valderrama J, Wilde P, Macierzanka A, Mackie A. The role of bile salts in digestion. *Advances in Colloid and Interface Science.* 2011;165(1):36-46. http://www.sciencedirect.com/science/article/pii/S0001868610001995. Accessed Nov 16, 2017. doi: 10.1016/j.cis.2010.12.002.

156. Dean W, English J. Medium chain triglycerides (MCTs) | nutrition review. . 2013.

157. Mahan LK. *Krause's food & nutrition therapy.* Saunders/Elsevier; 2008. Accessed Nov 16, 2017.

158. Armand M, Pasquier B, André M, et al. Digestion and absorption of 2 fat emulsions with different droplet sizes in the human digestive tract. *The American journal of clinical nutrition*. 1999;70(6):1096. http://www.ncbi.nlm.nih.gov/pubmed/10584056.

159. Shilling M, Matt L, Rubin E, et al. Antimicrobial effects of virgin coconut oil and its medium-chain fatty acids on clostridium difficile. *J Med Food*. 2013;16(12):1079-1085. Accessed Nov 18, 2017. doi: 10.1089/jmf.2012.0303.

160. Thormar H, Hilmarsson H, Bergsson G. *Antimicrobial lipids: Role in innate immunity and potential use in prevention and treatment of infections.* ; 2013:1488. Accessed Nov 18, 2017.

161. Gudmundur Bergsson, Jóhann Arnfinnsson, Ólafur Steingrímsson, Halldor Thormar. In vitro killing of candida albicans by fatty acids and monoglycerides. *Antimicrobial Agents and Chemotherapy*. 2001;45(11):3209-3212. http://aac.asm.org/content/45/11/3209.abstract. doi: 10.1128/AAC.45.11.3209-3212.2001.

162. Nair MKM, Joy J, Vasudevan P, Hinckley L, Hoagland TA, Venkitanarayanan KS. Antibacterial effect of caprylic acid and monocaprylin on major bacterial mastitis pathogens. *J Dairy Sci*. 2005;88(10):3488-3495. Accessed Nov 18, 2017. doi: 10.3168/jds.S0022-0302(05)73033-2.

163. Omura Y, O'Young B, Jones M, Pallos A, Duvvi H, Shimotsuura Y. Caprylic acid in the effective treatment of intractable medical problems of frequent urination, incontinence, chronic upper respiratory infection, root canalled tooth infection, ALS, etc., caused by asbestos & mixed infections of candida albicans, helicobacter pylori &

cytomegalovirus with or without other microorganisms & mercury. *Acupunct Electrother Res.* 2011;36(1-2):19-64. Accessed Nov 18, 2017.

164. Asprey D. *Head strong: The bulletproof plan to activate untapped brain energy to work smarter and think faster-in just two weeks.* HarperCollins; 2017. Accessed Nov 18, 2017.

165. Portalatin M, Winstead N. Medical management of constipation. *Clin Colon Rectal Surg.* 2012;25(1):12-19. Accessed Nov 18, 2017. doi: 10.1055/s-0032-1301754.

166. Christodoulides S, Dimidi E, Fragkos KC, Farmer AD, Whelan K, Scott SM. Systematic review with meta-analysis: Effect of fibre supplementation on chronic idiopathic constipation in adults. *Aliment Pharmacol Ther.* 2016;44(2):103-116. Accessed Nov 18, 2017. doi: 10.1111/apt.13662.

167. Müller-Lissner SA, Kamm MA, Scarpignato C, Wald A. Myths and misconceptions about chronic constipation. *Am J Gastroenterol.* 2005;100(1):232-242. Accessed Nov 18, 2017. doi: 10.1111/j.1572-0241.2005.40885.x.

168. Jetté M, Sidney K, Blümchen G. Metabolic equivalents (METS) in exercise testing, exercise prescription, and evaluation of functional capacity. *Clinical cardiology.* 1990;13(8):555-565. http://www.ncbi.nlm.nih.gov/pubmed/2204507. doi: 10.1002/clc.4960130809.

169. Nosrat S. *Salt, fat, acid, heat: Mastering the elements of good cooking.* Simon & Schuster; 2017. Accessed Nov 13, 2017.

170. Renwick AG, Molinary SV. Sweet-taste receptors, low-energy sweeteners, glucose absorption and insulin release. *British Journal of Nutrition*. 2010;104(10):1415-1420. http://journals.cambridge.org/abstract_S0007114510002540. doi: 10.1017/S0007114510002540.

171. Anton SD, Martin CK, Han H, et al. Effects of stevia, aspartame, and sucrose on food intake, satiety, and postprandial glucose and insulin levels. *Appetite*. 2010;55(1):37-43. http://www.sciencedirect.com/science/article/pii/S0195666310000826. doi: 10.1016/j.appet.2010.03.009.

172. Koyama E, Kitazawa K, Ohori Y, et al. In vitro metabolism of the glycosidic sweeteners, stevia mixture and enzymatically modified stevia in human intestinal microflora. *Food Chem Toxicol*. 2003;41(3):359-374. Accessed Nov 19, 2017.

173. Ukiya M, Sawada S, Kikuchi T, Kushi Y, Fukatsu M, Akihisa T. Cytotoxic and apoptosis-inducing activities of steviol and isosteviol derivatives against human cancer cell lines. *Chem Biodivers*. 2013;10(2):177-188. Accessed Nov 19, 2017. doi: 10.1002/cbdv.201200406.

174. Raynor HA. Can limiting dietary variety assist with reducing energy intake and weight loss? *Physiology & Behavior*. 2012;106(3):356. http://www.sciencedirect.com/science/article/pii/S0031938412001175. doi: 10.1016/j.physbeh.2012.03.012.

175. Gross-Loh C. *The diaper-free baby: The natural toilet training alternative*. Harper Collins; 2009. Accessed Nov 19, 2017.

176. Bauer I. *Diaper free: The gentle wisdom of natural infant hygiene.* Penguin; 2006. Accessed Nov 19, 2017.

177. Thomas DM, Martin CK, Lettieri S, et al. Can a weight loss of one pound a week be achieved with a 3500-kcal deficit? commentary on a commonly accepted rule. *Int J Obes (Lond).* 2013;37(12):1611-1613. Accessed Nov 19, 2017. doi: 10.1038/ijo.2013.51.

178. Thomas DM, Martin CK, Lettieri S, et al. Response to 'why is the 3500 kcal per pound weight loss rule wrong?'. *Int J Obes (Lond).* 2013;37(12):1614-1615. Accessed Nov 19, 2017. doi: 10.1038/ijo.2013.113.

179. Vazquez JA, Kazi U. Lipolysis and gluconeogenesis from glycerol during weight reduction with very-low-calorie diets. *Metab Clin Exp.* 1994;43(10):1293-1299. Accessed Nov 19, 2017.

180. Bortz WM, Paul P, Haff AC, Holmes WL. Glycerol turnover and oxidation in man. *J Clin Invest.* 1972;51(6):1537-1546. Accessed Nov 19, 2017. doi: 10.1172/JCI106950.

181. Exton JH. Hormonal control of gluconeogenesis. In: *Hormones and energy metabolism.* Springer, Boston, MA; 1979:125-167. https://link.springer.com/chapter/10.1007/978-1-4757-0734-2_7. Accessed Oct 28, 2017.

182. Westman EC, Mavropoulos J, Yancy WS, Volek JS. A review of low-carbohydrate ketogenic diets. *Curr Atheroscler Rep.* 2003;5(6):476-483. Accessed Nov 19, 2017.

183. Langfort J, Pilis W, Zarzeczny R, Nazar K, Kaciuba-Uściłko H. Effect of low-carbohydrate-ketogenic diet on

metabolic and hormonal responses to graded exercise in men. *J Physiol Pharmacol*. 1996;47(2):361-371. Accessed Nov 19, 2017.

184. McCleary SA, Sharp MH, Lowery RP, et al. Effects of a ketogenic diet on strength and power. *Journal of the International Society of Sports Nutrition*. 2014;11:P41. doi: 10.1186/1550-2783-11-S1-P41.

185. Helge JW. Long-term fat diet adaptation effects on performance, training capacity, and fat utilization. *Med Sci Sports Exerc*. 2002;34(9):1499-1504. Accessed Nov 19, 2017. doi: 10.1249/01.MSS.0000027691.95769.B5.

Made in the USA
Monee, IL
03 March 2022

92196735R10177